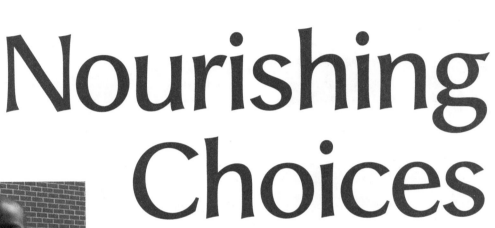

Nourishing
Choices

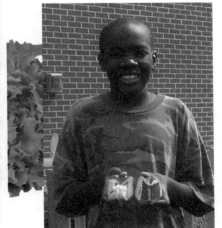

*Implementing
Food Education
in Classrooms,
Cafeterias, and
Schoolyards*

Eve Pranis

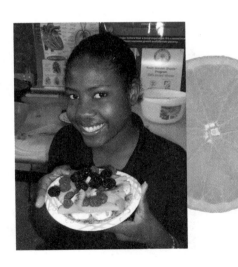

Published by the National Gardening Association
1100 Dorset Street, South Burlington, Vermont 05403 • *www.garden.org*

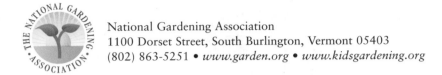

National Gardening Association
1100 Dorset Street, South Burlington, Vermont 05403
(802) 863-5251 • *www.garden.org* • *www.kidsgardening.org*

Founded in 1973, the nonprofit **National Gardening Association** (NGA) is dedicated to promoting home, school, and community gardening as a means to renew and sustain the essential connection between people, plants, and the environment. NGA's programs and initiatives highlight opportunities in five core areas: plant-based education, health and wellness, environmental stewardship, community development, and responsible home gardening.

Information. NGA disseminates horticultural information in a variety of forms — e-newsletters on a range of topics, books for educators and home gardeners, Web sites, and research — to promote gardening as a learning tool, a science, and an art. Learn more and subscribe to newsletters at: *www.garden.org/subscriptions.*

Grants. NGA administers a number of grant programs that award cash and products to schools and community organizations that actively engage youth in the garden. NGA also collects data to track the impact of these programs. For more information and to download applications, visit: *www.kidsgardening.org.*

Adopt a School Garden® (ASG). NGA's innovative program lets individuals and businesses establish or rejuvenate a school garden in their community based on their ability to help financially. Designed to link schools and youth gardens to donor funds, ASG directs and manages financial assistance, materials, and supplemental technical aid while providing ongoing support to the garden program. Learn more at: *www.garden.org/asg.*

Gardening with Kids Catalog. NGA's print and online catalog offers plant-based curricula, horticultural information, products that engage kids in active learning and exploration, and general items sized for young gardeners or designed to solve gardening challenges. Request a catalog or shop online at: *www.kidsgardening.org.*

National Garden Month®. Every year communities, organizations, and individuals nationwide celebrate gardening throughout April. Gardeners know, and research confirms, that nurturing plants is good for us: attitudes toward health and nutrition improve, kids perform better at school, and community spirit grows. Each year NGA offers a variety of projects and other ways for everyone to join the celebration. Learn more at: *www.garden.org/ngm.*

Printed in Canada.

ISBN-13: 978-0-915873-51-7

Library of Congress Control Number: 2008930319

Contents

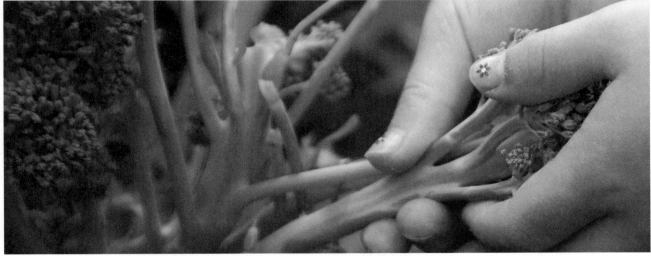

Foreword

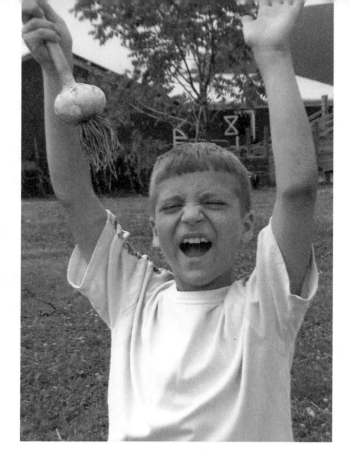

Consuming adequate amounts of fruits and vegetables is an important part of a nourishing diet, assisting in healthy child development, prevention of chronic disease, and weight maintenance.[1-8] However, less than 10 percent of American adults and adolescents consume the recommended amounts of fruits and vegetables.[9] Dietary patterns and preferences form in childhood and become habitual over time,[10] so helping children discover the joys of fruits, vegetables, and other whole foods sets the stage for a lifetime of healthier choices.

The Centers for Disease Control and Prevention estimate that the obesity prevalence in children and adolescents aged 6 to 19 tripled between 1980 and 2002.[11,12] This is an indication that young people are failing to develop a healthy relationship with the food environment, and change is needed now to prevent potential health problems. Schools provide a nearly universal opportunity to help turn this tide by providing a supportive and educational environment around the realm of food, which in turn may help young people eat better. *Nourishing Choices* is a resource outlining novel and systematic strategies for developing food education programs that get children excited about healthful foods, from schoolyard gardens and classroom cooking lessons to districtwide farm to cafeteria programs that bring local produce to the lunch line.

When children participate in gardening and in preparing and tasting foods, their familiarity with fruits and vegetables and willingness to try new foods improve with experience.[13-18] Students' consumption of fresh produce has been shown to increase when it is made available through farm to cafeteria arrangements.[19,20] *Nourishing Choices* synthesizes practices collected from successful programs that are using these tools and others to introduce children to wholesome foods.

Students gain much more from such experiences than good eating habits. In this book, the inspiring and illuminating stories of thriving programs reveal that combining complex concepts — food systems, sustainability and conservation, and community and cultural awareness — can engage children and help them see that health extends beyond their own bodies. Exposure to farms, hands-on gardening, and cooking all serve as introductions to systems thinking, giving children a real and holistic involvement with learning environments that integrate the sciences and humanities.

Nourishing Choices is a valuable tool for parents, educators, foodservice directors, school nurses, and nutritionists who are looking for ways to link health, academics, community, and the pure enjoyment of food from seed to plate.

Joel E. Kimmons and Terry O'Toole
Division of Nutrition, Physical Activity and Obesity
Division of Adolescent and School Health
Centers for Disease Control and Prevention

FOOTNOTES

[1] Hu FB. 2003. Plant-based foods and prevention of cardiovascular disease: an overview. *American Journal of Clinical Nutrition* 78(3): 544S-551S.

[2] Riboli E, Norat T. 2003. Epidemiologic evidence of the protective effect of fruit and vegetables on cancer risk. *American Journal of Clinical Nutrition* 78(3): 559S-569S.

[3] Glade MJ. 1999. Food, nutrition, and the prevention of cancer: a global perspective. American Institute for Cancer Research/World Cancer Research Fund, American Institute for Cancer Research, 1997. *Nutrition* 15(6): 523-526.

[4] Rolls BJ, Ello-Martin JA, Tohill BC. 2004. What can intervention studies tell us about the relationship between fruit and vegetable consumption and weight management? *Nutrition Review* 62(1):1-17.

[5] He FJ, Nowson CA, MacGregor GA. Fruit and vegetable consumption and stroke: meta-analysis of cohort studies. *The Lancet* 367(9507): 320-326.

[6] He K, Hu FB, Colditz GA, Manson JE, Willett WC, Liu S. 2004. Changes in intake of fruits and vegetables in relation to risk of obesity and weight gain among middle-aged women. *International Journal of Obesity Related Metabolic Disorders* 28(12): 1569-1574.

[7] Hung H-C, Joshipura KJ, Jiang R, et al. 2004. Fruit and Vegetable Intake and Risk of Major Chronic Disease. *Journal of the National Cancer Institute* 96(21): 1577-1584.

[8] Sargeant LA, Khaw KT, Bingham S, et al. 2001. Fruit and vegetable intake and population glycosylated haemoglobin levels: the EPIC-Norfolk Study. *European Journal of Clinical Nutrition* 55(5): 342-348.

[9] Kimmons JE, Gillespie C, Seymour J, Serdula M, and Blanck HM. U.S. Adolescent and adult fruit and vegetable intake at MyPyramid caloric requirement levels among a national sample. Under review. Centers for Disease Control and Prevention.

[10] Lake AA, Mathers JC, Rugg-Gunn AJ, Adamson AJ. Longitudinal changes in food habits between adolescence (11–12 years) and adulthood (32–33 years): The ASH30 study. *Journal of Public Health* (Oxford) 28:10–6.

[11] Ogden CL, Flegal KM, Carroll MD, Johnson CL. 2002. Prevalence and trends in overweight among U.S. children and adolescents, 1999-2000. *Journal of the American Medical Association* 288:1728-1732.

[12] Hedley AA, Ogden CL, Johnson CL, Carroll MD, Curtin LR, Flegal KM. 2004. Prevalence of overweight and obesity among U.S. children, adolescents, and adults, 1999-2002. *Journal of the American Medical Association* 291:2847-2850.

[13] Hermann JR, Parker SP, Brown BJ, Siewe YJ, Denney BA, Walker SJ. 2006. After-school gardening improves children's reported vegetable intake and physical activity. *Journal of Nutrition Education and Behavior* 38:201-202.

[14] Ozer EJ. 2007. The effects of school gardens on students and schools: Conceptualization and considerations for maximizing healthy development. *Health Education & Behavior* 34(6): 846-863.

[15] McAleese JD, Rankin LL. 2007. Garden-based nutrition education affects fruit and vegetable consumption in sixth-grade adolescents. *Journal of the American Dietetic Association* 107(4): 662-665.

[16] Graham H, Beall DL, Lussier M, McLaughlin P, Zidenberg-Cherr S. 2005. Use of school gardens in academic instruction. *Journal of Nutrition Education and Behavior* 37(3): 147-151.

[17] Demas, A. 1995. Food education in the elementary classroom as a means of gaining acceptance of diverse, low-fat foods in the school lunch program. Doctoral dissertation, Cornell University.

[18] Liquori T, Koch PA, Contento IR, Castle J. 1998. The cookshop program: Outcome evaluation of a nutrition education program linking lunchroom food experiences with classroom cooking experiences. *Journal of Nutrition Education* 30:302-313.

[19] Slusser W, Neumann C. 2001. Evaluation of the effectiveness of the salad bar program in the Los Angeles school district. School of Public Health, University of California, Los Angeles, cited in Farm to school: Strategies for urban health, combating sprawl, and establishing a community food systems approach. *Journal of Planning Education and Research* 23:414-423.

[20] Ralston K, Buzby J, Guthrie J. 2003. A healthy school meal environment. Food assistance research brief, USDA, Economic Research Service. Food Assistance and Nutrition Research Report (34-5).

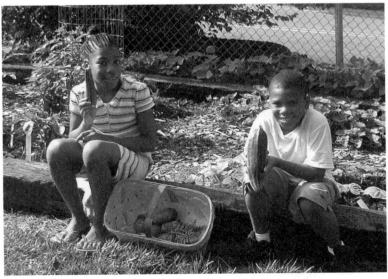

The findings and conclusions in this foreword are those of the authors and do not necessarily represent the official position of the Centers for Disease Control and Prevention

Acknowledgments

This book would not have been possible without inspiration and contributions from the following:

Bonnie Acker and Dan Treinis, Edmunds Middle School, Burlington, VT

Ashley Atkinson, Greening of Detroit, MI

Tammy Barron and James Fowler, Abernethy Elementary, Portland, OR

Barbara Berger, Las Cruces Public Schools, NM

Pepper Bromelmeier, USDA, Bellaire, MI

Timothy Cipriano, Local Food Dude LLC, Thomaston, CT

Linda Colwell and Kristy Obbink, Portland Public Schools Nutrition Services, OR

Diane Conners, Michigan Land Use Institute, Traverse City, MI

Trevor Davies and Eric Tompkins, Parks and Recreation, Wyoming, MI

Doug Davis, Burlington School District Food Service, VT

Ariel Demas, Hampstead Hill Academy, Baltimore, MD

Patti Evans, Isaac Dickson Elementary, Asheville, NC

Amy Gifford, Educational Consultant, Groton, MA

Dana Goodwin, Cori Oakley, and Tracey Westerman; Central Grade School, Traverse City, MI

Karen Heaton, Plainfield Elementary, NH

Emily Jackson, Growing Minds, Asheville, NC

Deborah Kane, Ecotrust, Portland, OR

Jeff Kessler, Central Lake, MI

Janet Miller, Buncombe County Schools, NC

Hope Miner, Kids Cook! Albuquerque, NM

Abbie Nelson, Vermont FEED, Richmond, VT

Stephanie Raugust, Pacific Elementary, Davenport, CA

Kevin Read, Richard Daley Academy, Chicago, IL

Clare Seguin, Lincoln School, Madison, WI

Jane Stacey and Lynn Walters, Cooking with Kids, Santa Fe, NM

Lisa Rose Starner, Mixed Greens, Grand Rapids, MI

Alisa Wright, Warren Elementary School, CT

Doug Wubben, Wisconsin Homegrown Lunch, Madison, WI

Thanks also to these experts for their thoughtful reviews and suggestions:

Amanda Archibald, R.D., Field to Plate

Melinda Hemmelgarn, M.S., R.D., Food Sleuth, LLC

Karrie Kalich, Ph.D., Keene State College

Mildred Mattfeldt-Breman, Ph.D., St. Louis University

Joel E. Kimmons and Terry O'Toole, Division of Nutrition, Physical Activity and Obesity; Division of Adolescent and School Health; Centers for Disease Control and Prevention

Photography

National Gardening Association

Front Cover (clockwise from top left): National Gardening Association (NGA), NGA, ©Dutto Davide/Dreamstime.com (tomatoes), Ariel Demas/Hampstead Hill Academy/Food Studies Institute, ©Bill Wolfe/Dreamstime.com (mixed fruit), NGA, Nathan Metallo, Dana Goodwin, NGA, ©Robert Milek/Dreamstime.com (mixed veg)

Back Cover: ©Robert Milek/Dreamstime.com (mixed veg)

Page 1: Nathan Metallo (top), Ariel Demas/Hampstead Hill Academy/Food Studies Institute

Fruits/vegetables throughout: ©Denis Pepin/Dreamstime.com (lettuce), ©Robyn Mackenzie/Dreamstime.com (orange), ©Boris Ryaposov/Dreamstime.com (tomato), ©Johannes Gerhardus Swanepoel/Dreamstime.com (yellow pepper)

Nourishing Choices Project Team

AUTHOR
Eve Pranis

EDITOR
Barbara Richardson

DESIGN & LAYOUT
Alison Watt

Introduction

Food looms large in young people's lives. But ask them to explain where it comes from, taste a vegetable-rich side dish on the lunch line, or discuss the cuisine of a culture, and they might be stumped.

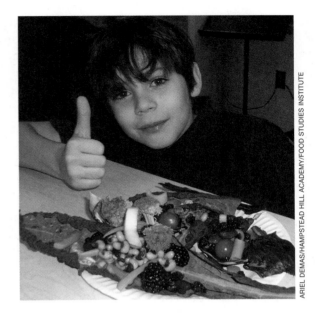

Add to that the fact that American children are heavier than ever and, as a result, at risk for a host of diseases. (The Centers for Disease Control and Prevention confirm obesity rates in those age 6 to 19 have more than tripled since the 1970s.) Despite such alarming statistics — and studies that link good nutrition to learning readiness, academic achievement, and decreased emotional problems — fat- and sugar-laden items continue to be part of the fabric of school life. Fresh fruits and vegetables are sorely lacking.

Now for the good news. Concerns about children's health, their disconnect from local food sources, and the persistent junk food "sell" that saturates their lives are fueling an appetite for change. In communities across the country, teachers, parents, community organizations, foodservice leaders, chefs, "lunch ladies," and farmers are bringing healthful foods and food education into classrooms, schoolyards, and cafeterias. These reformers contend that isolated nutrition lessons pack little punch when a child's environment sends conflicting messages, and that shifting eating behaviors takes more than knowing food facts.

Students are moving beyond memorizing minerals: They grow, cook, taste, and share plant-based foods and healthful dishes. Once hooked, youngsters become passionate advocates who help spread the word to others. As they savor the flavors and "life stories" of fresh local fare, they just might develop an enduring appreciation for what sustains us.

Many school-based food and nutrition projects are small-scale ventures initiated by teachers or parents: an indoor salad garden or wholesome weekly snacks made by students, for example. Others are multifaceted, involving a variety of school and community stakeholders who collaborate to hatch a sustainable plan for reforming the school food scene. Intrigued by the people we've discovered who are making nourishing changes — and by the experiences and advice they have shared — we created this book to support and inspire others.

How to Use this Book

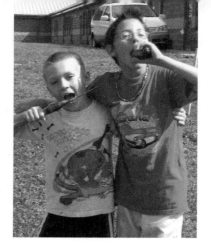

Nourishing Choices draws on a wealth of collective experience to help you develop a food education program and excite children about healthful eating. The first four chapters provide a roadmap for establishing your program. You'll discover what leaders who have paved the way for better school nutrition have learned about planning, finding support, and launching a workable program. Their "Fresh Ideas" and calls to "Take Action" are highlighted to help fuel your efforts.

Program Components

Project Profile	Page	Student Cooking Activities	Student to Farmer Connections	Student to Chef Connections	School Food Garden
Getting a Taste of Health	39	x			x
Kitchen Classroom	42	x			x
Harvest of Dreams	45	x			x
Food Education Curriculum Serves Up Sensory Lessons	48	x			
Nourishing School Fundraiser	52		x		
Homegrown Lunch	55		x		
Savoring Flavors in Las Cruces	58				
Appetizing Lessons in Kids Cook! Classrooms	62	x			
Good Things Cooking in North Carolina	64	x	x	x	x
Local Foods Rule	68		x		x
Shifting School Food Culture	73	x	x		
Lunch and Learning from Scratch	78			x	x

The profiles in Chapter 5 showcase a dozen exemplary projects that represent different contexts, designs, and entry points to better school nutrition education. The chart on these two pages provides a quick reference to elements highlighted in each profile.

The listings in Food Education Resources (Chapter 6) describe exemplary Web sites and print materials that can help you launch a new nutrition education program or strengthen an existing one.

Program Components, continued

Profile	Page	Farm to Cafeteria	Nonprofit Partner(s)	Multi-School or Districtwide	Specific Food Ed. Curriculum	Fundraising with Local Products
Getting a Taste of Health	39					
Kitchen Classroom	42				x	
Harvest of Dreams	45					
Food Education Curriculum Serves Up Sensory Lessons	48		x		x	
Nourishing School Fundraiser	52					x
Homegrown Lunch	55	x	x	x		
Savoring Flavors in Las Cruces	58	x		x	x	
Appetizing Lessons in Kids Cook! Classrooms	62	x	x	x	x	
Good Things Cooking in North Carolina	64	x	x	x		
Local Foods Rule	68	x	x	x		
Shifting School Food Culture	73	x	x	x		
Lunch and Learning from Scratch	78	x	x	x		

CHAPTER 1

Getting Started

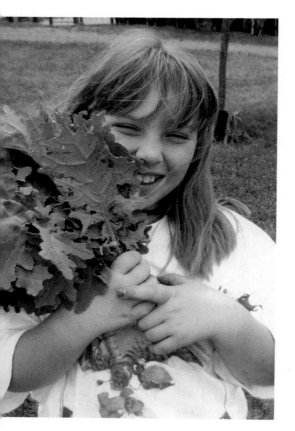

The impetus for shifting the school food environment can come from many places. Change might be driven by a school Wellness Policy or by an individual or group in the school, district offices, or outside community. Sometimes, a single — and apparently tireless — "champion" becomes a catalyst for change. But ventures with staying power more typically involve a variety of stakeholders who collaborate to bring a coherent food education vision to life. In the end, it takes a village: planners, passionate people who keep the ball rolling, those who state the case for change at the institutional and policy level, and young people who cook up solutions and educate peers, families, and the community.

Your entry point could be as straightforward as having kids grow salad greens or concoct healthy snacks. It could be as elaborate as an integrated farm to school program aimed at growing healthy bodies, minds, and local farm economies. In any case, you'll want to build alliances, start small, and test some ideas that you can build on.

Building a School Food Committee

Typically, two or more people concerned about children's health form a core food or nutrition committee or advisory group. They educate themselves, the school, and the broader community about the status of children's health, the school food "scene," and possibilities for change. As they do so, they invite others who have a stake in the process to help shape a vision, set goals, and develop an action plan. As the project evolves, the team develops a web of community partnerships that support the project at many levels.

The types of people who help launch school food projects — and those who become partners — are unique to each context. They frequently include the following:

School- and district-based individuals: Teachers, principals and other administrators; school board and PTO members; dieticians, nurses, and physical education and health instructors; guidance counselors; foodservice managers and staff; and students.

Community individuals and organizations: Parents; chefs; farmers; nutrition or gardening educators from Cooperative Extension offices; health professionals (e.g., nurses, dietitians, nutritionists, pediatricians); college faculty or graduate students; local or state health departments; government hunger or nutrition offices (e.g., federal child nutrition program); non-profit organizations working on community food, nutrition, hunger, agricultural education, gardening, or farm to school projects; food cooperatives, stores, or wholesalers; and local chapters of health organizations such as the American Dietetic Association and American Heart Association.

Assessing the Scene

If your committee's goal is to develop school food initiatives that meet genuine needs, it's important to gather relevant data. The information the team uncovers can also help you persuade potential funders, administrators, partners, parents, and participants of the need for — and value of — your proposed project. Answers to questions like these will fuel your work and planning:

– What does research say about issues like the link between school gardens and food choices, childhood obesity, and how nutrition affects learning readiness?

– What is the existing district or school Wellness Policy (see sidebar, p. 15)? Is it gathering dust or being used as a blueprint for change?

– How are teachers promoting good nutrition? What are their concerns? Who is most excited by the idea of teaching nutrition? (You can poll them via informal discussions or a paper or e-mail survey.)

– How comfortable are educators with teaching nutrition, preparing food with students, or using the garden as a learning tool?

– What is the status of the school's nutrition and health standards or curriculum?

– How nutritious is the food available to students in all school venues? What new foods and practices are likely to be most acceptable to students?

– Are foodservice staff members open to examining and testing some alternatives to the current practices? What limitations do they face? What new ideas and skills can they bring to the table?

– What are students' eating habits and preferences in the cafeteria? (Foodservice staff can help observe or measure them.) What changes would students like to see?

– What types of nutritional principles guide parents' food choices? What is their interest in learning about other options?

Nutrition educators and researchers report that isolated lessons are unlikely to persuade children to adopt healthy eating behaviors.

– What are the community's social and cultural norms and values regarding food and nutrition?

– Who else in the school system or community is taking action on similar issues? Is there an existing group with which to join forces (e.g., a local school health council)?

You can find links to helpful statistics and research in the Resources section of this book. You'll also find guidance for conducting a comprehensive assessment of school food and health policies and programs, as well as sample surveys, in these tools from the USDA and CDC:

✪ Changing the Scene: Improving the School Nutrition Environment: *www.fns.usda.gov/TN/Resources/changing.html*

✪ Comprehensive School Health Index: *http://apps.nccd.cdc.gov/shi/Static/paper.aspx*

Shaping a Plan: Questions to Spark Thought

Once your committee has a snapshot of the school food landscape and has identified people, organizations, and resources that can support your efforts, you can begin crafting a plan. Here we include some "big picture" questions and topical ones meant to spark thinking and discussion. For inspiration from the field, read the Project Profiles beginning on p. 39.

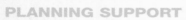

PLANNING SUPPORT

Here are two excellent planning tools for improving the school food environment:

School Foods Tool Kit (CSPI): *www.cspinet.org/schoolfoodkit/*

School Nutrition...by Design: *www.cde.ca.gov/re/pn/fd/ documents/schnutrtn071206.pdf*

"Big picture"
– What are our primary concerns and reasons for making changes in the school food and nutrition environment?

– What are our broad goals? What will it "look" like in the classroom, schoolyard, cafeteria, and community when our program is in full swing? (This is your long-term vision!)

– Given our assessment results, and the inventory of resources, which steps and strategies can we realistically tackle in this school year or the next one? How can we use these as stepping-stones to achieve our long-term vision?

– What will it take to get from here to there? Who do we need to involve in the process? Who will be responsible for what?

Stakeholders
– Who are the potential project partners and supporters in the school system and community? What are their concerns? Who might be resistant, and why? What types of appeals might pique their interest and prompt involvement?

– What types of alliances can help ensure the long-term sustainability of the initiative?

– How can we help staff, families, and the community reinforce the food and nutrition education messages?

– How can we represent the diversity of the district and community?

– How will we communicate with students, parents, and the broader community to solicit meaningful input from them?

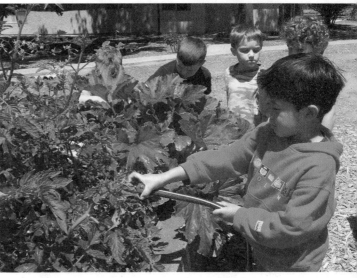

Student involvement

– How will we value students' voices and involve them in creating a healthy school food environment?

– How will we enable students to be advocates for healthful fare in the school and community?

– How will we engage students with local food and food producers?

School food and nutrition education

– What curriculum resources can we draw upon that support learning standards in all subject areas; encourage hands-on learning; and build knowledge, skills, attitudes, and behaviors that lead to healthful food choices?

– How can we integrate food and nutrition education outside the classroom (e.g., in the cafeteria, garden, after-school programs, special events, family homework materials)?

Professional development

– What forms of professional development would advance our school food initiative? Who could deliver them? (The focus might be helping teachers understand nutrition concepts and folding food education into the existing curriculum. It could also be helping foodservice staff procure, prepare, and cook fresh produce or new dishes.)

– Which types of print, electronic, or face-to-face forums can help participating students, faculty, staff, and partners exchange ideas, lessons, and experiences?

Food and nutrition policy

– What is the school's current policy for food and beverages available during the school day?

– Does our state legislature regulate any of this, or is it being discussed?

– Which nutritional guidelines would our committee and other stakeholders like to see implemented?

– What resistance might we encounter? What types of alliances can help move this initiative forward?

Evaluating the program

– How will we document progress toward our goals? (For example, will we look at the degree to which our project has (1) created a consistent schoolwide message about healthful eating, (2) increased student participation rates in a salad bar program, (3) reduced behavior problems, or

When students are engaged in planning, tasting, growing, cooking, or promoting new food choices to peers, they invest in the process.

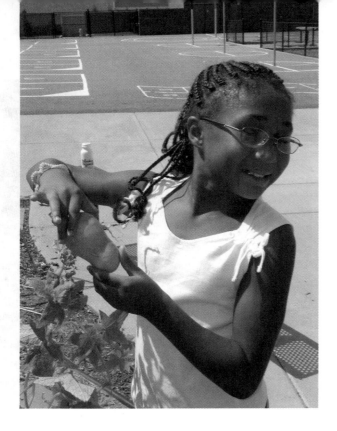

(4) influenced parents' nutrition knowledge and food choices?)

– What types of pre-evaluation/post-evaluation tools will help us document progress and secure future funding?

– How will we use our findings to further advance our efforts? How will we communicate them to school and community stakeholders?

Funding

– What is a viable budget for each component of our proposed project?

– How can we collaborate and leverage partnerships to find in-kind and financial support?

– What sources of funding and other support are available through the district, local agencies, businesses, the government, and local or national foundations?

Roles for partners

"You're only as successful as you are with your partners," says Ashley Atkinson, project manager at The Greening of Detroit. "Every community has a food bank, nonprofit food and educational organizations, nutritionists, and ties to universities. Be sure to identify clear needs when you approach a potential partner." Here are examples of the roles these allies can play:

⊛ Farmers, chefs, and other food producers visit lunchrooms and host field trips.

⊛ A chef or parent helps students make culturally relevant dishes.

⊛ A food coop cleans and prepares fresh produce for a healthy snack program.

⊛ A graduate student develops and helps implement standards-based curriculum modules for food education.

⊛ University faculty evaluate a garden-based nutrition project.

⊛ A grocery store donates dressings for a school salad bar.

⊛ A nonprofit hunger relief organization provides a VISTA worker to manage a school garden.

⊛ Master Gardeners from a state Cooperative Extension office facilitate an after-school food garden project.

⊛ A nutritionist hosts a workshop for teachers on integrating food and cooking activities into the curriculum.

⊛ A health insurance company sponsors a fresh food tasting project.

⊛ A nonprofit organization uses its public relations arm to alert the media about a district farm to school project.

⊕ A state legislator sponsors a bill that would help fund school nutrition gardens.

⊕ School board members develop a policy and nutrition standards for foods sold outside the cafeteria.

Obtaining Funds

What are you trying to fund? A monthly schoolwide taste-test event? A garden or farm to cafeteria project? A workshop for foodservice staff on preparing fresh produce? Be sure to involve your partners, business leaders, and other stakeholders (e.g., school board members) in seeking funding. Also look for ways to piggyback on their existing programs, staff, and resources. For instance, organizations might have funds earmarked for nutrition, gardening, or agricultural education. They might be able to place VISTA volunteers in your school or collaborate on proposals for grants that would otherwise be difficult to secure.

As you look for potential funders, be sure to consider these broad categories of interest: children's health, nutrition, and obesity prevention; food security and hunger; science and agricultural education; and sustainability of local farms. Here are some starting points.

Local businesses

It's good public relations to help youngsters thrive! Ask local businesses for cash or in-kind donations. Is a local coop willing to be a drop-off point for farm products or to prepare foods for a snack program? Approach a health insurance company about funding a taste-testing program. Be clear what your goals and needs are; when feasible, have students make the pitch.

Federal funding sources

The sources below support projects related to food, nutrition, and agriculture.

⊕ Food Stamp Nutrition Education Funds (*www.csrees.usda.gov/nea/food/fsne/progmap_text.cfm*): These funds are geared to schools in which at least 50 percent of students are eligible for free or reduced lunch. Some organizations have used the funds for cooking programs. The link goes to a list of state contacts.

⊕ USDA Child Nutrition Programs (*www.fns.usda.gov/cnd/Contacts/ StateDirectory.htm*): Ask your state coordinator about Team Nutrition school programs, materials, and mini grants.

⊕ Community Food Project Grants (*www.csrees.usda.gov/fo/ communityfoodprojects.cfm*): These funds support comprehensive

Take Action

SCHOOLWIDE NUTRITION AND WELLNESS POLICIES

The federal government issued a mandate through the Child Nutrition and WIC Reauthorization Act of 2004 to establish standards for diet and health in public schools. By 2006, each district was supposed to form a Wellness Committee and draft a policy that addressed nutrition education, physical activity, and nutrition standards for all foods available during the school day. Learn about your district's policy and discuss with administrators how to best put it into action.

Looking for inspiration or wording for a school-based policy? You will find links to sample policies in Resources, under "Planning."

projects that help communities become more self-reliant in meeting food and nutrition needs.

⊗ Sustainable Agriculture Research and Education Grants (*www.sare.org/grants/index.htm*): These have been used to support farmers' access to new markets, including farm to school projects.

⊗ School-Based Interventions to Prevent Obesity (*http://grants.nih.gov/grants/guide/pa-files/PA-06-417.html*): These grants encourage partnerships between school systems and academic institutions.

Other federal funding sources worth exploring include the National Science Foundation, Environmental Protection Agency, and U.S. Department of Education.

Private foundations (nonprofit or corporate)

Local community or education foundations typically provide start-up funds or support special projects within existing programs. Corporate foundations often fund programs in regions where they do business. These entities, along with regional and national foundations, have specific areas of interest. For instance, the Robert Wood Johnson Foundation currently "awards grants to combat childhood obesity by promoting healthy eating and physical activity in schools and communities." To identify funders and their interests, start with the resources listed below or consult a reference librarian.

Links to sources of funding

Loads of research exists that can help you state the case to potential funders for making a healthy shift in school food. These sites list current health-related funding opportunities available from federal agencies, private foundations, and businesses. You'll find other links in the Resources section.

⊗ The Healthy Youth Funding Database (*www.cdc.gov/HealthyYouth/funding/index.htm*)

⊗ SchoolGrants (*www.schoolgrants.org*)

⊗ The Center for Health and Health Care in Schools (*www.healthinschools.org/News%20Room/Grant%20Alerts.aspx*)

⊗ National Gardening Association Grants (*www.kidsgardening.com/grants.asp*)

Spreading the Word

Share your story, publicize your successes, and announce events! Getting the word out will help you gain outside support in the initial stages and sustain it over time. See it as an opportunity to recruit volunteers, attract new partners and funders, keep participants informed, and catalyze change in the broader community. Here are some ways to do this:

Take Action

FARM TO CAFETERIA SUPPORT

In June 2004, the Child Nutrition and WIC Reauthorization Act was passed, which includes farm to cafeteria legislation titled Access to Local Foods and School Gardens. The legislation aims to create a grant to cover the initial costs of farm to cafeteria projects. As of this writing, it has not been funded. Ask your legislators to help it move forward!

Develop a collection of materials to take on the road.
This could include program descriptions, handouts,
relevant statistics, newsletters, photos, videos, new
lessons, student work, a PowerPoint presentation,
or a Web site.

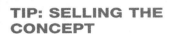

Find opportunities to present your story. Describe
how your school's story fits into a national movement. Here are some possible venues: community
health and nutrition events; professional conferences;
school board, PTA, or student council meetings; local or
state legislative sessions; meetings with potential partners
or funders.

Write articles or ask others to write them. Approach editors
at local newspapers and publications of community organizations or municipalities (e.g., American Heart Association
chapter, Chamber of Commerce). A school or community
leader might be willing to write an op-ed piece. Encourage
parents, teachers, students, and other advocates to write letters to the editor.

> ## TIP: SELLING THE CONCEPT
>
> Wondering how to inspire teachers,
> parents, administrators, and cafeteria
> workers to think about transforming
> school food? Serve them a stellar
> cafeteria-style lunch (plastic tray and
> pint of milk included), invite them to
> listen to compelling speakers talk
> about school food projects, and offer
> workshops on topics like cooking
> with kids and developing food and
> garden curricula.

When you pitch an idea for an article, radio spot, or op-ed piece — or try to
persuade a member of the press to visit you — come up with an angle that
will spark interest. Then try to paint a picture with your words. If you want
a journalist to come to your school, tie your invitation to an event such as a
nutrition garden dedication, special lunch featuring student-designed recipes,
or kickoff of a salad bar project. Be sure to have some brief written materials available: bullet points about your program, short vignettes, or a list of
supporting statistics or quotes about children's health.

Put together a mailing list. A mailing list should include community and
media people who are — or should be — interested in your project. Be sure
to include local radio and public access TV stations as well as journalists.
Send out e-mail or paper press releases about noteworthy project changes or
events. Follow up with phone calls to key people.

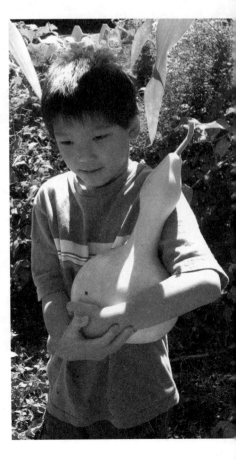

Have an event or celebration. This could be a global dinner, harvest festival,
or nutrition fair. Invite the media and local officials in addition to your
usual roster of partners and parents.

Now that you have a broad view of planning, remember the initial advice to
start small and build on your accomplishments. Your school's approach will
be unique to your situation and resources. Enjoy the adventure!

CHAPTER 2

Nurturing a Schoolwide Food and Nutrition Message

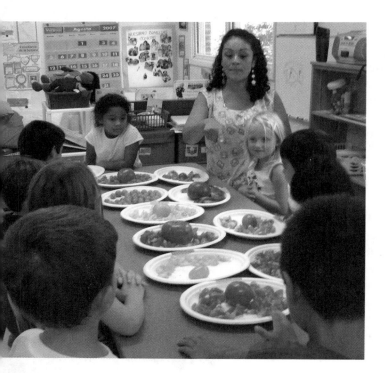

It's a familiar drill: Memorize the food pyramid or the rationale for eating greens. But nutrition educators and researchers report that isolated lessons are unlikely to persuade children to adopt healthy eating behaviors. Nor can kids easily counter conflicting messages from candy-based fundraisers, unhealthful vending machine choices, and free notebooks touting fast food. Then there's the sophisticated mass marketing that saturates students' lives outside of school. These all speak volumes about what's "desirable" to consume.

Organizers of the most effective school food and wellness initiatives acknowledge *all* the ways in which the school environment, directly and indirectly, teaches kids about food and health. Then they work toward sending a consistent message.

Best Practices

Leaders in school food and nutrition projects have a lot to say about setting the stage — in and out of the classroom — for a healthy lifelong relationship with food. Here we share some of their wisdom. You'll find more detail in coming chapters. Finally, you'll see how these strategies are put into practice in the Project Profiles.

Involve students as much as possible. When students are engaged in planning, tasting, growing, cooking, or promoting new food choices to peers, they invest in the process. When adults value their opinions and encourage them to pose solutions, young people become motivated, confident, collaborative learners. They plan gardens, market local foods, sit on food and nutrition committees, conduct taste tests, have a voice in vending choices, and come up with alternative fundraising ideas.

Don't ban or preach. Rather, invite again and again! "The underlying message we tend to send about nutrition in schools is that kids make bad (unhealthful) food choices and that we need to teach them what's good for them," says Luisa Peris of Italy's Slow Food in the Schools program. Instead of telling students what they shouldn't eat, or preaching about what's healthy, try to inspire curiosity and make discovering new foods irresistible!

Don't use food as a reward or withhold it as a punishment. This can undermine healthy eating behaviors. Eating nourishing foods should be seen as pleasurable, not as a bargaining chip. And using sweet treats as rewards for eating vegetables sends the wrong message about fresh fare.

Encourage adults to model good eating habits and the joy of sharing food. When teachers, administrators, staff, and parents join students for classroom snacks, school lunches, and school-based community meals, the adults have a chance to "walk the talk."

Work toward consistent food and nutrition messages in all school food venues. It is possible to shift traditions related to classroom snacks and parties, and to change the foods sold for fundraisers, at sporting events, in vending machines, and a la carte in the cafeteria. Some changes will be easier than others; administrative support is key. View this shift as part of a long-range plan.

Weave studies of food, food systems, and nutrition into the curriculum. Increasing demands tend to limit educators' willingness to take on so-called "extras." A committee or group of stakeholders can evaluate existing resources, look for overlaps with local learning standards and goals, and identify ways to use food and nutrition topics as learning themes or enrichment for core subjects. (For suggestions and tools, see Resources.)

Get parents and guardians on board. Build bridges to students' home lives by engaging and informing parents, and helping them model healthful eating habits. Here are some ideas:

⊛ Send home recipes or a newsletter with nutrition information, activities, and assignments that parents and children can do together: reading food labels, locating recipes, or conducting a kitchen scavenger hunt, for instance.

⊛ At a parent–teacher night or other event, set up a taste-test table or a display with recipes and photos of student chefs.

⊛ Host a special meal, fair, or festival for parents and other community members; have students help plan and prepare it.

⊛ Work with partners to offer workshops on preparing healthful snacks, buying and cooking with farm-fresh foods, and raising urban food gardens.

Fresh Idea

TIP: PYRAMID PARTIES

Third graders in Terra Bella Elementary in California employ a unique food twist for classroom parties. Instead of consuming sweets, the class plans and prepares snacks by drawing from one or more of the healthful food groups on the food pyramid. Word has it that the cheese, cracker, and fruit theme was "awesome!"

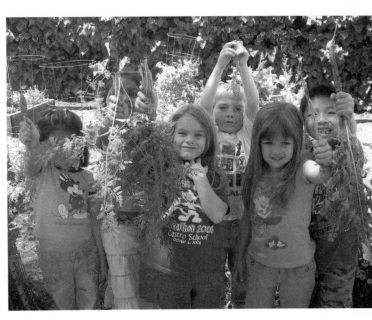

✥ Invite parents to volunteer in the garden, chaperone farm field trips, or run cooking sessions to share special recipes with students.

✥ Send home seeds and seedlings to inspire home gardens.

Use the cafeteria as a classroom. Be sure to enlist the skills and perspectives of the foodservice staff, and to respect the limitations they face. Showcase foods, tasting activities, and presentations or materials from student gardeners, chefs, nutritionists, and local farmers. Create time, opportunities, and an aesthetic environment for students to relish foods and the social aspect of sharing meals. (Also see Chapter 4, Transforming the Lunchroom Experience, page 32.)

Involve community partners. Each school and community has a unique mosaic of people and organizations with an interest in children, community health and nutrition, gardening, cooking, cultural exchange, or sustainable farm economies. By engaging and drawing on these groups, you will enrich and find support for your efforts. Equally important, you will enable students to interact with a host of people of different ages, cultures, and socioeconomic status who are passionate about healthful edibles.

Extend food and nutrition education beyond the school day. After-school cooking or gardening programs, student-run community food events, and family food projects can reinforce your message and broadcast it to the larger community.

Grow it! The word is out. When students have a hand in growing food themselves, they are more willing to eat it. A full-blown school garden might be impractical, but even a few pots of tomatoes or a window-box salad garden can give students a chance to nurture and sample fresh food.

Encourage students to share food with others in the community. Hold a community harvest festival or international dinner, perhaps tied in with history, geography, and peace studies. Or bring school garden goods or student-made foods to a soup kitchen; older students can interview people there to explore why they need assistance.

AFTER SCHOOL WITH PARKS AND REC

A federal 21st-Century Community Learning Centers grant helped the Parks and Recreation department in Wyoming, Michigan, work with partner Mixed Greens to deliver a winning after-school project. For 45 minutes four days a week, at-risk students and those new to the urban school grow foods, create healthful snacks (such as pumpkin soup and fresh salads), and plan and prepare a family dinner. (Slow cookers and other portable cooking gear make it possible.) Says recreation programmer Trevor Davies, "Parks and Rec departments don't just dribble basketballs; this type of program fits their mission, and their organizational strength looks good to potential funders."

Core Components

What does a school that is committed to nurturing a better food environment "look" like? There are many answers! But exemplary programs seem to include at least some of the following core activities.

Tasting sessions

When students have opportunities to experience new flavors, describe them, and state preferences, they are more likely to opt for new foods in the cafeteria and elsewhere. If they've grown or prepared edibles themselves, even better.

If you tackle tasting sessions on a large scale, discuss and plan the project with foodservice staff. Ask local farmers or food stores to donate items for tasting events or ask local funders to underwrite food costs. Here are a few twists on the theme:

✿ Hold classroom taste tests using fresh garden or farm produce. Have students describe each item's characteristics: appearance, flavor, texture, and aroma. They could compare items (e.g., types of melons or tomato varieties) and rank their preferences, sample a vegetable or fruit prepared in many different ways, or compare locally grown items with store-bought counterparts.

✿ Hold a "Taste of ____" event while studying another country or historical era. Feature music, stories, and cultural items (e.g., chopsticks) along with samples of relevant dishes crafted by students and adult volunteers.

✿ Before introducing a new snack or lunch item, invite students to try a bit and share opinions. Peers can dish it up and then survey diners. Renee DeWindt, foodservice director in Benzie County, Michigan, performs her taste tests survivor-style. The question she puts to students: "What should survive to the next menu?" Be sure to use student input to make decisions about menu changes.

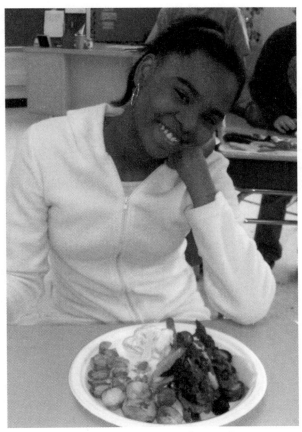

ARIEL DEMAS/HAMPSTEAD HILL ACADEMY/
FOOD STUDIES INSTITUTE

Cooking opportunities

Give students good ingredients and a little guidance and watch their confidence and openness to new flavors bloom. In this era of convenience foods, young people need opportunities to experience the ritual and pleasures of co-creating and sharing cuisine.

✿ Prepare healthful snacks in class at least once a week.

✿ Invite local chefs, parents, or nutrition educators to cultivate young cooks. Use a school, restaurant, or community organization kitchen, or bring cooking carts, slow cookers, electric frying pans, or other portable equipment into classrooms. (Be sure to check school fire codes first.) Give the adults tips on how to communicate with your class's age group and which foods are most practical for them.

✿ Start an after-school cooking club. Your recipes don't have to require lots of labor or equipment. Pickle garden produce, make salsa or veggie-topped pizzas, design fresh fruit kebabs, or create interesting salads or smoothies.

✿ Have students and volunteers produce a community meal or a harvest or health festival with food sampling stations.

✿ Hold a cook-off or meal in which students taste and describe what they like about other families' recipes or cuisine from different cultures.

...try to inspire curiosity and make discovering new foods irresistible!

Visits to local food businesses

Arrange student visits to farms, farmers' markets, specialty food producers (e.g., cheese makers), restaurants, food coops, and community supported agriculture (CSA) farms. Let the hosts know your project's goals and what you hope students will gain from the visit. Prepare students by exploring how the producer or business fits into the local food system, community, and economy.

On a farm visit in Central Lake, Michigan, fourth graders got a taste of community economics along with farm-raised snacks. The grower posted a chart representing people who worked on the farm. She used it to explain how the farm income also supports other workers and businesses in the community.

School gardens

There's something about planting, nurturing, and harvesting peas, carrots, radishes, arugula, and other garden trophies. It makes fruits and vegetables worth tasting! In fact, research studies point to the value of school gardens for increasing students' nutrition knowledge and preferences for fruit and vegetable snacks.

A plot full of edibles can also inspire students to try creative classroom cuisine; explore foods and growing techniques from other cultures, past and present; or uncover the life stories of particular food crops. It can push students to think beyond their own food choices and work toward improving nutrition and stemming hunger in their communities. Here are a few ways to link gardens to nutrition education:

⊛ Grow food-themed garden plots: pizza or salsa, Asian or Mexican foods, the "three sisters" (corn, beans, squash), the food pyramid, and so on.

⊛ Set up a cafeteria compost project or otherwise explore decomposition and its relationship to plant and human nutrition.

⊛ Make garden-inspired snacks: salads, vegetables with dips, roasted pumpkin seeds, carrot soup. Also use garden items to supplement school lunches.

⊛ Conduct taste tests of different fruit varieties or compare garden-grown items with store-bought counterparts.

⊛ Plan a harvest festival. (See Harvest of Dreams, page 45.)

⊛ Create a garden-inspired community meal, such as a stir-fry supper.

⊛ Sell fresh garden items or processed ones (e.g., pickles, salsas) at a community or school farmers' market. Provide nutrition information on labels or brochures.

Take Action

GARDENS NOURISH KIDS — STATE THE CASE

Teachers and parents everywhere concur: When kids grow fruits and veggies, they eat them! These anecdotal reports are supported by a recent study showing that adolescents who participated in a garden-based nutrition intervention increased their servings of fruits and vegetables more than in a non-gardening nutrition education group. You'll find links to related research under Resources (p. 84).

(McAleese, J.D., and L.L. Rankin. 2007. Garden-Based Nutrition Education Affects Fruit and Vegetable Consumption in Sixth-Grade Adolescents. **Journal of the American Dietetic Association.** *107(4): 662-665.)*

Farm to school learning connections

Farm to school programs give local farmers a reliable demand for their products, bring fresh foods into classrooms and cafeterias, and enhance student nutrition. Just as important, such programs help students develop personal connections and agricultural literacy that can lead to an enduring preference for local edibles. Chapter 4, Transforming the Lunchroom Experience, discusses the logistics of the farm to cafeteria concept. In addition to visiting local farms, as discussed on the previous page, here are some other strategies for connecting students to the people and practices behind the foods they consume.

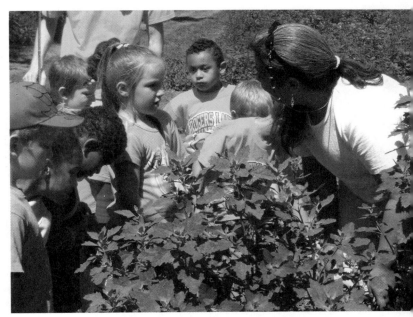

Bring farmers into school. As part of Wisconsin's Homegrown Lunch project, each school is assigned a designated "farmer/educator." In addition to visiting classrooms, the growers attend special school events and host class field trips. At some schools in Portland, Oregon, when a local "harvest of the month" item is featured, the grower greets students in the lunch line and attends a "meet the farmer" question-and-answer session during recess. You can also invite local growers to participate in a school harvest festival.

Make a cafeteria or hallway display titled Who Produces Our Food? Post photos, letters, graphs, and stories featuring local farms and food providers.

Alternative fundraisers

School fundraising programs are a multibillion-dollar industry that tends to peddle foods low in nutritional value. The products selected often contradict a school's other health and wellness messages. But kids don't have to push candy to raise a buck. You can help them invest in the local community and good health by offering a different twist on food. Sell these types of items or services during special school market days or via a pre-order system:

⊛ Thematic vegetable or fruit baskets or boxes

⊛ Vegetable or herb seedlings or flower bulbs

⊛ Locally produced foods (e.g., cheeses, fruit jams, honey, breads, herbs)

⊛ Fruit and yogurt parfaits

⊛ A student-created healthy foods cookbook

⊛ Tickets to a harvest supper or meal representing the community's cultural groups

⊛ Walk-a-thon entries

⊛ Garden-based crafts (e.g., potpourri, pressed flower stationery, herbal soaps)

☺ Bagged compost or mini worm bins

Try to offer items grown or made by students, farmers, and local businesses. You can read about such a venture in the Nourishing School Fundraiser profile, page 52.

Schoolwide food themes and events

Focusing the entire school on a food-themed event is a good way to engender excitement, reinforce learning, and build community. Here are some sample events:

☺ Annual harvest meal or local foods dinner

☺ A cook-off with healthful family recipes

☺ Edible "celebrity" vegetable or fruit of the month or farm harvest of the month (see Sample Project, below)

☺ Fruit and vegetable festival complete with fruit and salad bar, costumes, music, and learning games

☺ Global dinner with dishes from one or more cultures represented in the curriculum or community

☺ Fruit and vegetable market

☺ Healthful snack cart (Students prepare foods to sell during school breaks or after school)

☺ Nutrition and fitness theme at an open house.

Sample Project: Edible Celebrity of the Month

Make a splash by focusing on a new healthful item each week or month. Set this up as a classroom, team, grade level, or schoolwide venture. Enlist support from the foodservice staff or from parent or community volunteers. Here's some advice from the field:

Choose a featured food or category. Be sure to include items that are in season in your region or locally available. (Check the school garden first!) Fruits and vegetables are ideal, but you could also choose a type of locally made cheese or bread, or a food from another region (e.g., Middle Eastern dips).

Decide how to prepare the food. Perhaps you'll make and serve an item in different ways (e.g., raw apples, applesauce, apple muffins, and carrot–apple salad). If the celebrity food will be served in the cafeteria, be sure to involve foodser-

Fresh Idea

TIP: HEALTHFUL ITEMS FOR SNACKS, CELEBRATIONS, VENDING MACHINES

When selecting snacks, look for organic options and those without excess packaging.

Fruits: Whole, sliced, canned, frozen, or dried items; fruit salad, applesauce, fruit kebabs and dips (e.g., strawberries in yogurt); fruit pops; low-sugar fruit rollups, fruit smoothies (with yogurt, milk, or juice)

Vegetables: Raw items with low-fat salad dressing or other dips (hummus, bean dip, salsa), veggie pita pockets or wraps, salads

Grains/Nuts: Whole-wheat English muffins or pita bread, whole-grain crackers, rice cakes, baked tortilla or pita chips, whole-grain cereals, cereal bars, trail mix, soy nuts

Dairy: String cheese, low-fat yogurt or cottage cheese with toppings, yogurt smoothies, kefir

Drinks: Water, seltzer, low-fat milk or soy milk, 100 percent fruit juice (plain or mixed with seltzer)

vice staff in planning. Can they use help preparing the food? How will it be served?

Seek donations from local growers, food suppliers, or stores. Find out if a representative is willing to come into class or host a field trip. (A business or foundation interested in children's health might also be willing to cover food costs.)

Decide how to involve students. Collaborate with art, science, and English teachers. Students could research the celebrity food and create hallway or cafeteria displays complete with cool facts, photos and artwork, nutritional highlights, recipes, and growing information. They could also schedule taste tests for the school community. Ask students to think about what they want to find out and how they will gather feedback. For instance, they could create oral or written surveys that ask tasters to rate the food's appearance and flavor. Generate broader publicity for the celebrity item by having students take home recipes, create a newsletter for parents, or prepare and serve food samples at an open house.

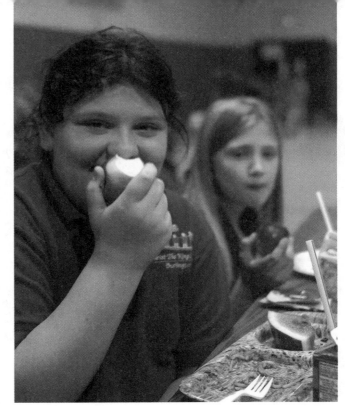

NATHAN METALLO

Extend the learning. Take a trip to a local market garden or farm to see the featured food growing. Calculate the number of miles this food would travel to reach your school's cafeteria, and compare this number to the miles the food travels when sourced through typical channels. Explore how to grow the item organically. Uncover its origins and related folklore. Find out how the food is used and how it is regarded in different cultures.

Beyond lunch: shifting other school food practices

The United States Department of Agriculture regulates the nutritional value of foods that are part of the federal school meals program. But there are few limits on the sale of foods and beverages offered a la carte in the cafeteria and in school stores, vending machines, sports events, and other school venues. (These are called "competitive foods" because they compete with the federal program.) No surprise: Soda and sports drinks, salty snacks, candy, and high-fat baked goods make up the bulk of goods served and sold as competitive foods.

Administrators and PTOs have traditionally seen vending contracts, which are often exclusive, as vital sources of funds for the school. In reality, the big companies benefit *much* more than schools do. In fact, soda companies have worked hard to block state legislation banning soda sales in schools!

But across the country, countless schools have switched to selling healthier foods — and banned unhealthy ones altogether — without losing revenue.

"The school system is where you build brand loyalty."
— John Alm, former president, Coca-Cola
Atlanta Journal Constitution, May 5, 2003

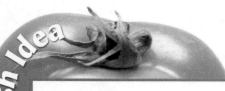

Fresh Idea

RECIPE CONTEST BOOSTS CAFETERIA CHOICES

In the ConVal district in New Hampshire, students sharpened their skills during a recipe contest for school meals. They were invited to submit recipes that followed specific guidelines for nutrition, portion size, and pricing. Proud concocters saw their meals (such as "Real Deal Nachos": multi-bean chili with veggies and homemade chips) served as part of a monthlong showcase of student recipes.

(Adapted from Going Local: Paths to Success for Farm to School Programs, *by the National Farm to School Program and others.)*

Nutrition committees have created policies that outline which categories of foods are and are not acceptable. Some schools have negotiated with vendors to test healthier options. Some state legislatures have passed bills to regulate competitive foods. In the end, students have accepted changes, *especially* when they have been tapped for suggestions or feedback. (You can read about model programs on this Web site: *http://teamnutrition.usda.gov/Resources/ makingithappen.html.*)

Soda companies are taking notice. In May 2006 the American Beverage Association signed an agreement with the Alliance for a Healthier Generation to improve their product offerings to schools. Visit *www.healthiergeneration.org* for more information.

CHAPTER 3

Connecting Food Education to the Curriculum

Your school's subject-area standards, instructional philosophy, and unique context will influence how your food and nutrition focus intersects with the curriculum. One strategy is to use food- and nutrition-related content and experiences as a central theme for learning across the curriculum. Or use them to supplement and enrich learning in different disciplines or in just one core subject (e.g., science or health).

Planning

Consider convening a curriculum selection or development group consisting of educators who wear different hats: a curriculum specialist; health, nutrition, or gardening teacher; and science coordinator, for instance. Invite someone from a partner organization (e.g., a nutritionist) to join the committee or provide lessons or materials for your group to review. You should already have gathered information on teachers' attitudes, experiences, and concerns about food education.

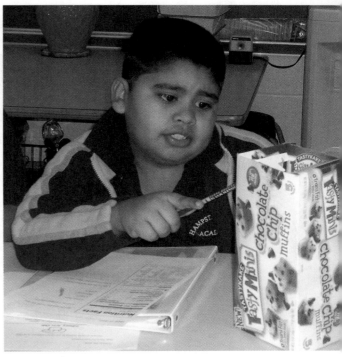

ARIEL DEMAS/HAMPSTEAD HILL ACADEMY/
FOOD STUDIES INSTITUTE

Loads of curriculum materials covering gardening, food systems, and nutrition are available online and in print (see Resources). Try to review and evaluate some of what's out there so you can decide which to use or adapt and what to create yourselves.

Next, ask, "What is important for students to learn about food, food systems, and nutrition? What's the best way to teach it?" Remember that food education experiences can also help meet broader goals of a school or district in such areas as learning readiness, character education, obesity prevention, multicultural learning, and civic responsibility.

As you gather and develop instructional resources, think about how you will solicit and incorporate teacher input; manage materials; and provide instructional, technical, and moral support.

Best Practices

What types of learning environments prepare students to be curious, thoughtful food consumers? This list of best practices from the field can inform your program.

⊛ Instruction supports experiential inquiry-oriented learning that cultivates curiosity and openness to new food experiences.

⊛ Students apply math, science, and literacy skills through activities such as cooking, gardening, and "marketing" foods to peers.

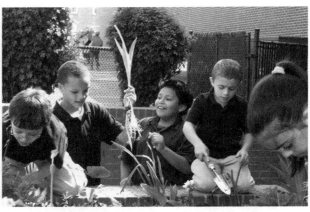

ARIEL DEMAS/HAMPSTEAD HILL ACADEMY/
FOOD STUDIES INSTITUTE

⊛ Learning experiences build conceptual understanding, skills, attitudes, and behaviors that promote healthful food choices; they also help students apply learning to real-life situations.

⊛ The curriculum enables students to learn about food systems (local and global) and the social and cultural aspects of food.

⊛ Educators help learners make connections among the classroom, garden, cafeteria, and community.

⊛ Students explore their own experiences, opinions, and values related to food and nutrition, and they share these with others.

⊛ Multiple food-related events and contexts support learning goals (e.g., school fundraising, classroom parties).

⊛ Some learning takes place out of the classroom (e.g., during recess, lunchtime, or after school), especially if there are constraints on classroom instruction time or methods.

⊛ Students have opportunities to teach others (for instance, older students plan and present an interactive lesson for a younger class, or develop materials for a family health fair).

⊛ Parents and other community resources are involved in ways that reinforce curriculum goals.

⊛ Pre- and post-assessments document the benefits of the program.

Teacher Support

Teachers need adequate time, materials (e.g., cooking or gardening equipment, lesson plans), and instructional support for teaching about food and nutrition. This is most likely to happen when such lessons are part of a schoolwide health and wellness program. Here are some ways to get started:

"Package" some lessons. Encourage nutrition committee members, partners, or subject area teachers to develop or adapt relevant kits, lessons, or thematic modules. Make time for teachers to review or field-test lessons and provide feedback. Give them a chance to experience the lessons as learners or see them modeled.

A science teacher at Huntington Beach Union High School in California created five nutrition-related science labs in "ready-to-go kits" for other science teachers. (In one, for example, students burned a potato chip and measured its calories.) The kits featured lesson plans and chemicals for experiments and food samples from the foodservice department!

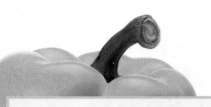

Match support to teachers' needs. Do teachers want to see examples of how classroom cooking or ethnic theme gardens can help meet core subject standards? Learn basic nutrition information? Experience garden investigations as learners? Co-plan lessons with a nutrition specialist? See a food systems lesson modeled?

Once you know what teachers want, find people who can help deliver support, such as nutrition educators, chefs, and other district and community resource people. Their interaction with teachers could occur via inservice workshops, collaborative teaching sessions, or lunchtime meetings.

Facilitate teacher collaboration. Encourage colleagues to co-plan and share lessons, resources, and challenges with one another and with nutrition committee members. They could do so through an after-school inservice session, a bulletin board, a student-catered lunch, a district conference, an online chat room, or e-mail.

Ideas for Enhancing the Core Curriculum

Involving students in food-related experiences naturally supports the nutrition and health curriculum. It also offers a real-life context for growth in personal development (e.g., making healthy choices), civic responsibility (raising public awareness about local food issues), and social skills (collaborating to cook, garden, or create surveys). But it's the core disciplines that remain on the hot seat, so below you'll find some sample teacher-tested curriculum ideas for these subjects.

Language arts and media

Communication skills flourish when students have a compelling context for employing them. Consider these approaches:

⊛ Use food tasting to help students stretch their senses and descriptive skills. For example, encourage them to describe something as "peppery" or "zesty" rather than "yucky." In doing so, they expand their openness to new flavors and their abilities to describe them.

⊛ Keep food or garden journals or diaries.

⊛ Use children's fiction and nonfiction books or poems as starting points for exploring foods, gardens, farms, and nutrition (for instance, Pablo Neruda's *Ode to Tomatoes*). Teachers in the Pajaro Valley district in California met with the children's specialist at a local bookstore to select relevant titles.

Once you know what teachers want, find people who can help deliver support, such as nutrition educators, chefs, and other district and community resources people.

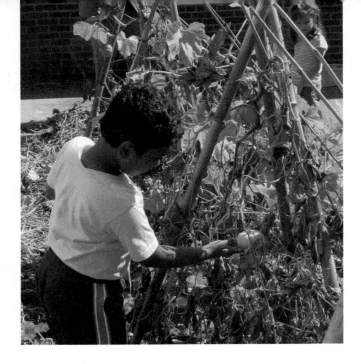

- ✺ Create a classroom or school cookbook of recipes inspired by local garden or farm items, or by cultural cuisines of your community.

- ✺ Create a public service announcement or an advertising campaign promoting fruits and vegetables, a healthful cafeteria offering, or a food-related event.

- ✺ Analyze the many influences on our food intake and choices: family, friends, culture, emotions, sensory stimuli, and marketing. Critically examine strategies used by the food industry to promote low-nutrient food products.

- ✺ Interview and photograph growers at a local farmers' market and create a multimedia presentation for the school community.

Math

Math becomes practical and relevant when students conduct these types of activities and apply concepts learned in the classroom:

- ✺ Design and grow gardens. Plan, measure, plant, and calculate compost needs.

- ✺ Cook. Weigh and measure ingredients, multiply recipes, convert measurements from U.S. units to metric ones.

- ✺ Peddle plant products. Calculate expenses, prices, and net income for a school market or fundraiser.

- ✺ Design a cafeteria food preference survey and then gather, represent, and analyze data.

- ✺ Visit a supermarket and find out where selected produce items originated. Calculate the relative distance that each travels from where it's grown to the lunchroom. Compare that to the distances traveled by locally grown counterparts.

Science

School gardens, farm visits, cooking sessions, and food studies offer countless possibilities for "real-world" science. As students pursue intriguing questions, they use their senses and reasoning and communication skills to make sense of the world. Here are some examples of food-related science activities.

- ✺ Explore physical and chemical changes of foods during cooking. (See "Thematic Lessons" in Resources.)

- ✺ Compost waste from cafeterias, cooking projects, and gardens. Make connections between food waste, decomposition, and plant and human nutrition.

- ✺ Research ways to grow tomatoes and then try some. Gather, represent,

When students have opportunities to experience new flavors, describe them, and state preferences, they are more likely to opt for new foods in the cafeteria and elsewhere.

and analyze data to find out which method produces the largest (or tastiest) fruits.

☺ Try to list the environmental costs and benefits of eating local foods versus those that travel great distances to our tables. Then conduct some research. (Do the same for "sustainable" versus "conventional" food, farming, or gardening systems.)

Social studies

Food and plants have influenced — and been influenced by — human cultures and societies. Here are some ways students can delve into these connections:

☺ Discover why local foods rule! (See "Thematic Lessons" in Resources.)

☺ Research the histories of foods in lunch boxes, school gardens, farm fields, or farmers' markets. Discover where the plants originated, the impact they've had on our diets, and how they've been used by different cultures across time.

☺ Interview parents, grandparents, and community elders about changes in foods eaten or plants grown during their lifetimes; culturally important recipes; special gardening techniques; plant or food folklore; memories of plants used for celebrations; and medicinal uses of specific plants.

☺ Compare cultural food preferences. Have students from different backgrounds keep lists of all the plants they eat in a week. As they compare lists, discuss observations and work together to answer questions that emerge.

☺ Grow foods or use gardening techniques from another culture or time period. Discover through folklore how and why people valued different types of plants and planting systems. For instance, research and plant a Native American "three sisters" garden (corn, beans, and squash) or an Asian planting.

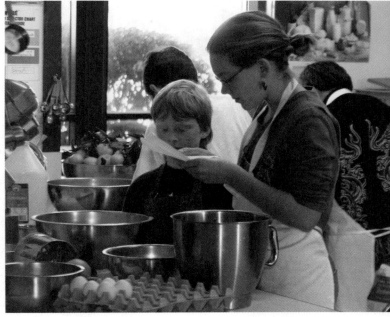

ALICIA DICKERSON/LIFE LAB

CHAPTER 4

Transforming the Lunchroom Experience

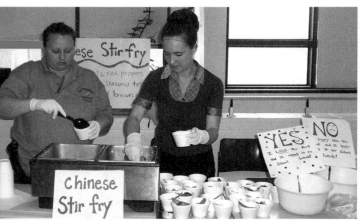

ARIEL DEMAS/HAMPSTEAD HILL ACADEMY/
FOOD STUDIES INSTITUTE

The phrase *school lunch* once conjured up images of mystery meats and scoops of pale produce. But at least it was made in the school kitchen! Over time, cafeteria cuisine got a bit of a makeover. After all, schools lose money when kids don't buy lunch. Kid "comfort foods" became standard fare in many lunchrooms. The trouble is, many of these favorites are fatty, high in sugar, and devoid of fresh fruits and vegetables. The disconnect between the health lessons students learned in the classroom and those they absorbed in the lunchroom was hardly a surprise!

A Menu for Change

But things are shifting, driven largely by concerns about obesity and children's health and by federal requirements for school wellness policies. Here's a glimpse of what's afoot in cafeterias across the country:

Students are participating. They set up taste tests, state preferences, survey peers, help create menus, collaborate with cooks, and "market" new foods to the school community.

Cooks are adjusting old favorites. Think whole-wheat pizzas with low-fat cheese and vegetable toppings, or baked — rather than fried — fries. Some foodservice managers have even gotten vendors to modify items made off-site. Students appear to be fine with the changes, if they notice them at all.

Students have access to more fresh, local, and international foods. Farm to cafeteria programs are flourishing. Kitchen employees are also serving up new dishes that showcase plant-based foods and reflect the cultural diversity of communities.

Image matters! Kitchen staff and nutrition committees are attending to the visual appeal of foods and to the aesthetics and social aspects of the lunchroom environment.

Cafeterias are serving as classrooms. Menus highlight nutrition connections. Farmers proffer tastes of produce and related lessons. Students post photos, art, and other displays touting the benefits of eating local foods.

In the end, say those working to transform school food, kids are eating — and savoring — new foods and flavors.

Sounds great. But trying to alter lunchroom content and culture can be a slow process fraught with personal, political, financial, and logistical hurdles. It is beyond the scope of this chapter to dig deeply into these issues. However, leaders of school food projects throughout the country have been testing and evaluating new ideas, and their lessons can help fuel your efforts. You'll find inspiration and advice in the Project Profiles, and excellent online and print materials in Resources. In the rest of this chapter, we touch on what advocates of school food change have learned about getting foodservice staff, students, and local farmers on board.

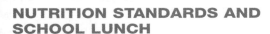

NUTRITION STANDARDS AND SCHOOL LUNCH

The National School Lunch Program requires that meals meet certain nutritional standards, but it doesn't regulate foods sold a la carte in the cafeteria (or elsewhere in the school). Moreover, many nutritionists say the guidelines aren't stringent enough. Many schools have begun to set their own nutrition standards for foods served on campus. A raft of current and pending legislation promises to smooth the way for healthful and farm-fresh lunchtime fare. (See the School Nutrition Association Web site for policy updates: *http://capwiz.com*.)

Healthful Liaisons: Working with the Foodservice

Across the country, advocates of transforming school meals echo the same refrain: Involve the foodservice directors and staff. Recognize the limitations they face *and* the ideas and expertise they bring. Work toward incremental — not dramatic — shifts in the lunch scene.

Shifting gears with school food can be tricky, in part, because our National School Lunch Program has traditionally prioritized cheap foods over more health-enhancing options. Free and low-cost government commodities run heavily toward fatty cheeses, meats, and processed items. Foodservice managers cite these types of challenges in incorporating fresh — particularly local — items:

☻ Seasonality and expense of fresh produce

☻ Local growers' inability to meet demands of large schools or districts

☻ Extra labor time and costs required for preparation

☻ Lack of training in preparing and cooking from scratch

☻ Logistics of local procurement, delivery, and storage

☻ Getting central kitchens or outside vendors to incorporate new or fresher foods

☻ Requirements that schools purchase from food vendors with liability insurance (which small-scale farmers don't typically carry)

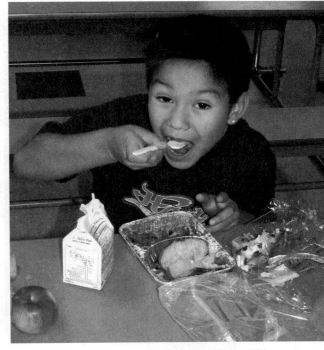

WISCONSIN HOMEGROWN LUNCH

✿ Meeting the bottom line

A note on the final challenge: Most foodservices must be self-supporting, so directors need to sustain high sales, and many assume they have to appeal to kids' appetites for low-nutrient foods. However, initiatives from California to Maine reveal that students will actually opt for healthful foods, as long as they're tasty and kid friendly!

Despite some trepidation, many foodservice workers have a passion for food and a commitment to nourishing children. They *know* that what's being served isn't great. Concerned directors nationwide, buoyed by local Wellness Policies, are ripe for change. Alliances between foodservice staff, farmers, and local food advocates or nutrition committees are prompting creative shifts and impressive results. Here are suggestions from advocates who have successfully collaborated with foodservice personnel.

Involve foodservice staff on nutrition committees. They should help create — or at least be privy to — the "big picture" of a changed school food landscape. Learn about their constraints and work together to brainstorm solutions. Solicit recipe suggestions and ideas for creating excitement in the cafeteria: a grand opening of a "fruit salad station," monthly taste test, or café-like decor.

Help the foodservice identify relevant training opportunities. A chef or state foodservice employee might help cooks tweak recipes to include more fresh items or use more healthful government commodity foods (e.g., dried beans).

Encourage staff to get their feet wet by making small changes. This could include a few food theme days (e.g., global lunch, farm-fresh harvest, pumpkin fest), a student taste test of a potential menu item, or healthy eating tips on menus and displays. Staff might also contribute recipes and nutrition information to a school Web site or cafeteria menu.

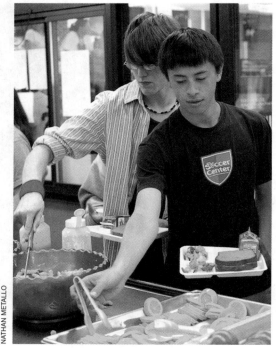

Help foodservice directors network with others. Put them in touch with farm to school programs and other organizations that can state the case for change and provide resources, services, and funds. (Go here to see if there's a program in your state: *www.farmtoschool.org.*)

Unfortunately, many school kitchens are sorely lacking in equipment, including sharp knives! In many places, stoves have given way to holding ovens for reheating foods. In an ideal world — and perhaps in the future — districts would have funds to invest in full kitchens along with better-paid and -trained employees. More realistic short-run alternatives to improving meals include giving cold dishes a nutritional boost, using holding ovens in new ways (for instance, for roasting vegetables), and having central or satellite kitchens, commissaries, or vendors make wholesome recipes.

NATHAN METALLO

Hooking Students and Tantalizing Taste Buds

When students are involved in selecting, preparing, tasting, and rating foods — and discover that their opinions and preferences are valued by the foodservice or snack program coordinators — they are apt to become invested in the process and products. They, in turn, become committed consumers, advocates, and "salespeople."

All the components discussed in Chapter 2 help students become more receptive to new foods and flavors. Here are some more ways — specific to the cafeteria — to engage and involve them.

Invite students to form or sit on a school food advisory committee. Young members can share insights, suggestions, and preferences related to cafeteria offerings. You can also assemble a temporary student delegation to give input on a proposed lunchroom feature such as a sandwich bar.

Survey cafeteria customers. What do students like and dislike? What new healthy foods would they like to see? How much did they like a taste-test item? Would they eat it again? Students are more likely to respond if their peers ask the questions directly or via a survey. Results were encouraging when high school students in Burlington, Vermont, asked what new foods diners would like to see: ethnic/international foods, less mayo, a fresher salad bar, and more baked and grilled items to replace fried ones! (See profile on page 73.) Present results to the student body, administration, foodservice manager, or other group. Use student feedback to inform menu changes.

Plan creative promotions. In Olympia, Washington, the school foodservice first introduced organic salad bars at school assemblies and then brought a "traveling salad bar" into classrooms.

Whet students' palates. Have a parent or school gardener bring a new food item into classrooms each week or month, introduce it, and engage students' taste buds. (If you have facilities, students can cook or otherwise prepare it.) *Then* feature the same item or recipe in the cafeteria.

Pass out samples in the lunchroom or set up a taste-test table. Better yet, have students do this. These sessions could feature new vegetables and fruits, familiar ones served in new ways (e.g., green beans drizzled with ranch dressing), or samples of a potential new menu item. Follow up with an interest or preference survey.

Have students "sell" the idea of fresh or healthful foods. Challenge a small group to develop a marketing campaign for local produce, a new salad bar

Take Action

PLENTIFUL PICKINGS AT THE SALAD BAR

Efforts to boost the nutritional value of school meals often begin with salad bar projects. (A UCLA study in a low-income neighborhood found that adding a salad bar to the cafeteria, where students could choose their own fruits and vegetables, increased produce consumption at lunch by 40 percent.) Some are once-a-week ventures; others are permanent lunchroom features. Fresh fruits and produce — often from local farms and school gardens — tend to be the mainstays. They can be accompanied by dairy products, breads, and healthful protein sources such as sunflower seeds, nuts, and other toppings. On page 86, you'll find resources for launching a salad bar program. (Find a summary of the UCLA study here: *http://dailyhealthfeed.com/school-lunch-fruits-vegetables*.)

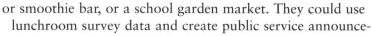

SQUAPPLE FOR ALL

Chef Timothy Cipriano (aka The Local Food Dude) gave recipes using locally grown products to middle school consumer science students. They did a cost and nutritional analysis of each recipe, then prepared a small version to sample in class. Next, students "marketed" the dish to the school community. Later that week, Timothy prepared enough for all cafeteria goers to try. The most popular recipe was Squapple, a winter squash and apple crisp with a cornflakes topping! (See *http://localfooddude.com*.)

or smoothie bar, or a school garden market. They could use lunchroom survey data and create public service announcements, skits, bulletin boards, posters, or other persuasive presentations.

In addition to promoting the idea within the school, students can learn to advocate for broader policy changes such as funding for farm to school programs. For instance, they might write letters to the editor, present their ideas to the school board, or call in to radio shows.

Invite students to help develop menus or recipes. Working in small groups, your budding chefs will have to learn how nutritional guidelines work and use math skills to create meals and menus that comply.

Make it attractive. Half the allure of eating is the visual appeal of food and the environments in which we consume it. Ask a local chef to conduct a session for kitchen staff on cooking, garnishing, or presenting appetizing dishes. Invite art classes to come up with creative labels for food packages (e.g., wraps) or paintings of fresh-picked produce. Some foodservice staffs have even transformed the eating space to look like a café or international market.

In this era of convenience foods, young people need opportunities to experience the ritual and pleasures of co-creating and sharing cuisine.

Showcase the people behind the food! Post displays or menus that feature photos of growers and their farms along with highlights of their operations and, if appropriate, sample products. Also invite producers to meet students in the cafeteria, classrooms, or an after-school club.

Feature foods that support lessons or health themes. An Indian meal and spice-tasting session could wrap up a study of the subcontinent. Whole-wheat rolls could follow a unit on dietary fiber. An all-apple lunch day (Waldorf salad, squash and apple soup, apple crisp) could complement a week of related studies or a farmer-in-the-classroom event.

Set up a cafeteria composting operation. As youngsters participate, they'll make connections between the cycle of decomposition, regrowth, and health: School lunch waste enriches soils, which in turn grow wholesome foods that help us thrive. Consider composting with worms!

Use printed or online menus to draw in students and parents. Highlight cooking techniques, cool cultural and historical facts about menu items, nutrition information, recipe links, food humor, and the producers who provided ingredients.

Ask for feedback. Feature a suggestion box or area in the cafeteria where students can state opinions and preferences for current items or suggest new ones.

Hook families, too! Invite them to eat in the lunchroom regularly or on special meal days. Routinely send a newsletter home that describes lunchroom changes, highlights the program goals, and features recipes and nutrition information. Set up taste tests for parents during open house or parent–teacher conference nights.

Farm to Cafeteria: The Promise and Challenge of Fresh Foods

At its best, improving the school food environment means forging lasting connections with farmers and other local food sources. After all, local produce is more nutritious. The riper a fruit is when it's picked and the sooner you eat any produce after picking it, the more nutrients it contains. But there are other reasons to seek out food grown close to home. Bringing farm goods to school helps kids make fruitful connections to growers and helps them understand their food's roots and routes. Kids also eat more produce when it's fresh from the farm. You'll find links to research studies in Resources.

Farmers win, too. Connecting with cafeterias gives them a reliable market at a reasonable price. (Farmers typically receive only 10 to 20 cents of every dollar consumers spend on food. The rest goes to pay for packaging, transportation, processing, and marketing!) In the end, when schools use foods produced closer to home, students' taste buds and bodies flourish, along with the health of local farms and rural economies.

The basics of farm to school

In farm to cafeteria programs, schools and districts buy directly from growers or farm cooperatives, local farmers' markets, local food wholesalers, or the Department of Defense Fresh Fruit and Vegetable program (see Resources). A variety of stakeholders typically collaborate to address the challenges that each scenario presents as well as the concerns. For instance, how do you efficiently and cost-effectively procure and transport adequate quantities of foods from a variety of sources, store them, and ensure that they're processed and ready for cooking?

Partner organizations, such as food coops, might lend support such as providing storage space or labor for cleaning and cutting snack items. Some farmers form cooperatives to facilitate distribution and make items kitchen-ready. The start-up costs and extra labor needed to incorporate fresh farm foods tend to be high, but so do teacher and student participation rates in the program (and thus income). School chefs committed to using local plant-based foods have found ways to pare back

FINDING COMMON GROUND

Both teachers and foodservice staff at Summerville Elementary School in California were concerned about students' eating habits and wasted food. With this common concern, they asked the local Cooperative Extension Service (CES) to provide a joint workshop. As an "outsider," the CES agent was able to present information that everyone at the workshop accepted. As a result, cooks and teachers came up with creative, concrete ways to improve students' nutrition awareness and food choices. Students were surveyed about their favorite foods, and they now help design menus. The CES agent helped the staff fit favorites into menus in ways that met nutrition standards. The agent was so impressed by the collaboration that she and her staff got more involved with school gardens and cooking!

(Adapted from Strategies for Success II: Enhancing Academic Performance and Health Through Nutrition Education, *by the California Department of Education.)*

other costs or bring in extra income (for instance, by cutting back on desserts or catering staff meetings).

The best farm to school programs also provide training or otherwise help foodservice personnel incorporate more fresh produce in ways that entice and nourish kids. And they integrate educational components in the classroom, cafeteria, and curriculum.

Resources for getting started

Intrigued? Find out if there's a farm to school program in your state by checking out *www.farmtoschool.org*. Then start small by working with that group — or another agricultural partner — to identify a grower or several who can supply one or more seasonal farm items in adequate quantities for a seasonal recipe or meal. In Portland, Oregon, for instance, a side dish of local roasted squash is the district-wide entry in a Harvest of the Month program. Local apples, which require little preparation, go to school in droves in New Hampshire.

For other inspiration and guidance, read the Project Profiles starting on the next page. The online guide *Eat Smart–Farm Fresh*, from USDA's Food and Nutrition Service, is one of the best resources we've found on buying and serving fresh local foods in school meals: *www.fns.usda.gov/cnd/Guidance/ Farm-to-School-Guidance_12-19-2005.pdf*

FARMERS' COOP DELIVERS

Since 1995 the New North Florida Cooperative — covering Florida, Georgia, Alabama, Mississippi, and Arkansas — has grown, processed, and delivered farm-fresh produce for school meals. Participating farmers learn that selling "value added" products to school districts creates a long-term market that will help them capture a high price for their products. The group processes the produce so it's easy for kitchen staff to prepare — for instance, by washing collards and cutting sweet potatoes into sticks.

(Adapted from Going Local: Paths to Success for Farm to School Programs, *by the National Farm to School Coalition and others.)*

Getting a Taste of Health

I t started out as a week of wacky vegetable events during National Nutrition Month (March). "As part of our healthy eating focus, we'd hold a 'fruit and vegetable boogie,'" says school nurse and health educator Karen Heaton of Plainfield, New Hampshire. In preparation for the dance, K–8 students at Plainfield Elementary School dressed up as their favorite produce — for instance, salads or cauliflowers — and teacher deejays spun vegetable-themed tunes. Later, the whole school got to sample the real stuff. Karen and staff solicited donations from grocery stores and set up a free edible-themed snack table in the hallway. ("Exotic fruits" were a hit.)

> **Nutrition Committee Makes Inroads**
>
> Parents and staff form a school nutrition committee, assess the school nutrition environment, and find funding for a monthly food-sampling program.
>
> **Plainfield Elementary Plainfield, NH**

But Karen knew that shifting students' attitudes about greens and such — and their inclination to try them — takes more than a week of food frolic. With visions of a more sustained focus, she invited staff and parents to collaborate on a school nutrition committee. Their charge: To oversee and recommend positive changes to improve the school's nutrition environment. "Our main focus was on exposing students to healthy foods and teaching them how to incorporate them into daily food choices," explains Karen.

Savoring Garden Goods

The link between gardening, exercise, and nutrition was a no-brainer. So the committee secured grant funds to enable students, parent volunteers, and other community members to expand an existing schoolyard plot. Second and seventh graders planted together in the spring. Come fall, the same students harvested the bounty. In between, teachers used the site for drawing, journaling, measuring, and exploring science concepts.

But the real proof was in the tasting. With their harvest in hand, students set up a hallway display to showcase it for the school community. Next, they worked with nutrition committee members to prepare healthful recipes for a special "feast day." The school has no kitchen, but a local church group offered use of its facility. On the appointed day, proud eighth graders doled out samples of corn chow-

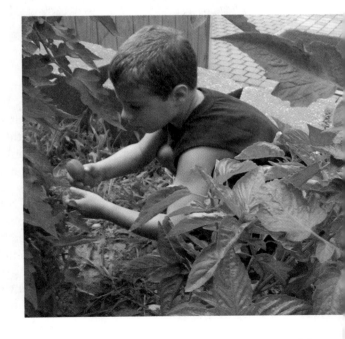

der, minestrone soup, zucchini pizza, cherry tomatoes with vinaigrette, and other garden-inspired treats to the rest of the school community.

The garden goods samples were such a success that the committee secured a state Team Nutrition grant to fund a sampling event each month of the school year — and to involve more students in the process. One month the student council prepared oatmeal and brought samples to each class. Another time, fourth graders worked with parents and staff to prepare and serve strawberry and yogurt parfaits. Sometimes a discussion of health benefits, or a questionnaire, would be served up along with the food. "We would conduct simple written surveys to see if the students liked the foods," says Karen. Some items — like chicken tetrazzini and minestrone — got so many thumbs-ups that students asked if the dishes could go on the lunchroom menu. It didn't hurt that the foodservice director had joined the committee. A little research revealed that the food vendor would be willing to produce a requested meal if it was feasible.

As students were priming their palates, their parents were receiving a weekly newsletter article from the nutrition committee. Along with food and nutrition information, the piece featured a question-and-answer column from a character called Nutricia.

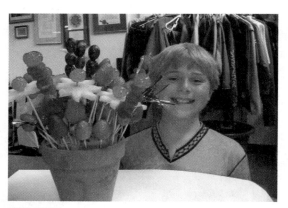

KAREN HEATON

Nutrition Committee Strategy: Assess, Plan, Promote

"Involving students in the process is key," explains Karen. No foods were banned or mandated, but her young charges are now apt to choose more wholesome lunch and snack foods. "We discourage unhealthy choices, but focus more on exposing students to healthy options," says Karen. And staff members make a big deal when students opt for those. For instance, when a fifth-grade boy brought a homemade flower pot filled with a fruit arrangement to school, that was a cause for celebration and a photo shoot!

"An effort like this takes a lot of work," Karen advises. "So make sure to involve others who share your passion; the more support, the better off you'll be!" But she suggests first doing some preliminary research. Before applying for the Team Nutrition grant, staff members and a parent used an assessment tool to get a read on the school's nutrition environment (see Assessing the Scene, p. 41). Then they presented the results to the nutrition committee. (When students and school board members later joined the group, it was renamed the Health and Wellness Council.) "It opened our eyes about how well we were doing on everything from nutrition education to vending machines," explains Karen. "It also pointed out our weak areas and gave us some tools for tackling those."

The assessment helped the committee develop a federally mandated Wellness Policy, which they posted on the Web site and presented to parents, school

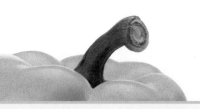

board members, and other stakeholders. Over the course of a year, the group incorporated feedback. Finally, they put together a related Health and Wellness Resource Guide for parents. According to Karen, the discussions sparked by the new policy made a tangible difference. "Parents are trying hard to think about what foods they send in for school celebrations and athletic events. Even school fundraisers have shifted tone. The Student Council now sells citrus fruits, and we carry only 100 percent juices and water in vending machines."

ASSESSING THE SCENE

The assessment tool used at Plainfield Elementary School drew from two comprehensive online resources: (1) The "improvement checklist" in Team Nutrition's tool kit, *Changing the Scene: Improving the School Nutrition Environment: www.fns.usda.gov/TN/Resources/ changing.html* and (2) The Centers for Disease Control and Prevention's Comprehensive School Health Index: *http://apps.nccd.cdc.gov/ shi/Static/paper.aspx.*

Kitchen Classroom

You won't find students in Stephanie Raugust's Davenport, California, classroom poring over textbooks. Instead, groups of fifth and sixth graders spend each morning cooking up fresh fare from scratch, laying out lunchroom tables, and serving the school community, family style.

"So many schools have centralized cooking and foodservices," says Stephanie. "But that removes everyone from the process." She doubts that students can grasp nutrition when it's simply presented in the classroom. Nor does she see much practical nutrition education in the science or health curriculum. In her opinion, food preparation and the social aspects of eating need to become a routine part of students' lives. After all, she notes, "We're up against a complex system in which big businesses make money marketing food to young people."

Stephanie's passion for introducing students to fresh foods and teaching them lifelong skills for healthy eating inspired what Pacific Elementary dubbed the "Food Lab" project 20 years ago. Over time, traditional prepackaged processed school meals gave way to more local menus that excited students' palates as they nourished the school community.

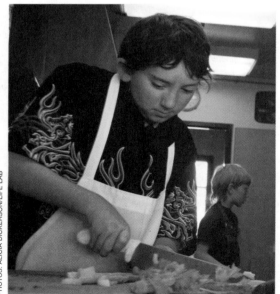

PHOTOS: ALICIA DICKERSON/LIFE LAB

Managing Cooking Teams

Stephanie works with a multigrade 5/6 class for two years. Each student cycles through the kitchen one morning a week, working with four to six peers. Tasks are clearly defined, restaurant-style: manager, baker, prep person, and cook. The manager must count the number of students eating lunch that day and calculate the amount of food needed. The baker measures ingredients and helps make the dessert. The prep person cleans and cuts the fresh foods, many of which come from local farms and the school's Life Lab garden. And the cook works on the main dish. Over time, as her young charges take on more responsibility, Stephanie steps back and advises. "After two years with a group of students, I can stand in the middle of the kitchen and watch students work on their own," she explains. "It's really something to see how well they all manage."

Spicing Up the Curriculum

Stephanie helps students connect what they do in the kitchen on a given day to key concepts and skills that support teachers' learning goals. Skills and concepts in math and more come to life, of necessity, as students plan and execute well-balanced meals. "We also play culinary games like exploring food-related language," says Stephanie. (*Don't be a couch potato; spice up your life!*) "Students find it entertaining, and it also helps them develop a respect for food and the culinary arts as a profession." Several of her students have indeed gone into the field.

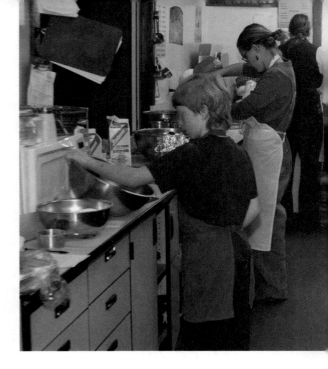

Come spring, each seasoned chef must develop a unique menu — with help from his or her cooking group — and produce it for the lunchroom crowd. Family favorites and cookbook recipes inspire student creations. There are, of course, some ground rules. For instance, meals need to meet state nutrition guidelines for relative quantities of protein, grains, and other nutrients. And Stephanie must be able to find ingredients or substitutes.

"It's become such a tradition that students anticipate the project well in advance," says Stephanie. After all, the name of the day's head chef is featured on the menu. And some meals are so popular that they live on. Take the year a student created a stuffed potato with cottage cheese and other nutritious ingredients. "I never would have thought of the combination, but now it's a standard menu item," says Stephanie.

Students in the kitchen classroom have a unique opportunity to become responsible, confident leaders as they prepare good meals for their community. In doing so, they develop lifelong skills that can help them and others thrive. Just as important, notes Stephanie, is their concrete and growing understanding of where food comes from and how you get it. "They see the produce guy — or farmer — bring in raw ingredients, and begin to make connections."

Then there are the less tangible social connections and lessons digested in the lunchroom. "The kitchen is the focal point in most homes," says Stephanie. She notes that Pacific Elementary's lunchroom plays that same role. Everyone — adults and students — eats together at tables set by the young cooks. Adults model good manners and openness to new items, and prompt food-related discussions.

Advice and Challenges

Stephanie admits that her program is feasible largely because she teaches in a small public school (100 students) with a principal who values hands-on learning of real-life skills. "It took a big buy-in for the administration to include much of my salary in the general budget and to consider my teaching role." She muses about how larger schools might give students a taste of the kitchen. "Students could prepare just one portion of a meal, such as a

> *It's... hard knowing in your heart what kids are gaining, but needing to find ways to document their skills and understanding.*
>
> — Stephanie Raugust, Pacific Elementary School, Davenport CA

daily fresh salad or soup, or they could shape rolls from dough that is already prepared." Kitchen staff might also invite a small group to tackle a project just once a month, rather than making it a daily or weekly event.

Even with administrative support, Stephanie faces other hurdles. "Government commodity foods tend to be cheap, but many, such as peanut butter, are high in sugar and fats." Purchasing more healthful alternatives can strain the budget. The good news is that on average, a whopping 80 percent of students — and many staff members — buy the school lunch. And that begins to make the finances of buying fresh, often local, foods more reasonable. That is, if you can find an efficient way to get produce from the farms to school. Stephanie suggests contacting regional farm to school programs or local produce wholesalers who, in some places, have begun to deal with area growers.

"It's also hard knowing in your heart what kids are gaining, but needing to find ways to document their skills and understanding," says Stephanie. "I think if you look at what our school spends and what it gets back, it is a worthy program." Evidently, others think so, too. Loads of parents say they chose the school because of its reputation for cultivating confident cooks and gardeners.

The School Garden Connection: From Seed to Table

Pacific Elementary's lunches are more than just tasty and good for you. Many of them feature the results of students' fruitful work in their Life Lab garden. Students working in the Food Lab plan the variety and amounts of green goods to grow, learn about food "seasons" in the garden, and preserve items they've harvested for later use (e.g., by drying beans).

During weekly garden visits, small student groups tackle a short science, nutrition, or team-building activity from the Life Lab curriculum, *The Growing Classroom*. Then they dig into their plots. Each group tends its own 5- by 10-foot raised bed that's bursting with salad greens, herbs, and other edibles earmarked for the Food Lab program. The young stewards harvest, clean, and package their goods before delivering them to Stephanie and their peers in the kitchen.

But it's not *all* about work. Students also have time to explore the garden each week on their own. They might forage in the food plots, take vegetables home, or wander through the labyrinth-like flower garden. As they do so, their curiosity and conversation spark new ideas for science and culinary investigations.

Harvest of Dreams

I magine this scenario: You stumble into the school cafeteria expecting yet another serving of tuna boats, but instead you find bare single-serving pizzas. Next, you're invited by other students to select your own toppings — but they're a bit unorthodox: sautéed squash, okra, eggplant, and other organic items from your school's garden. Much to your surprise, they taste great! Welcome to the Warren Elementary School's fall harvest luncheon.

When sixth-grade teacher Alisa Wright; her principal, Paula Cassidy; and students in Warren, Connecticut, first hatched the idea of a schoolyard community garden, they wanted it to be a vehicle for "making connections to food and to the environment, community, and curriculum." Now more than five years later, it's well on track. One of their secrets: Cultivate enthusiasm for garden edibles in the cafeteria and classrooms!

Making Pizza and More with Fresh Garden Themes

A school garden program builds leadership skills and inspires an annual student-led community harvest luncheon and cooking events.

**Warren Elementary
Warren, CT**

A Multigrade Alliance

The whole school is involved in what they dubbed the Harvest of Dreams garden, but it's the sixth graders who lead the way. These senior garden stewards are responsible for coordinating planning and planting each spring, teaching schoolwide garden lessons, and preparing and hosting their signature Harvest Luncheon in the fall.

Before planting time, Alisa's students develop lessons on such topics as sowing and composting. Then they spend 40 minutes in each classroom — dressed up as carrots and other edible characters — engaging and teaching garden helpers. Teams of the preteen leaders reinforce the concepts by taking youngsters into the garden for real-life demonstrations and practice.

Students and parents work on summer garden maintenance and bring early pickings to a local soup kitchen and food bank. Come harvest season, each

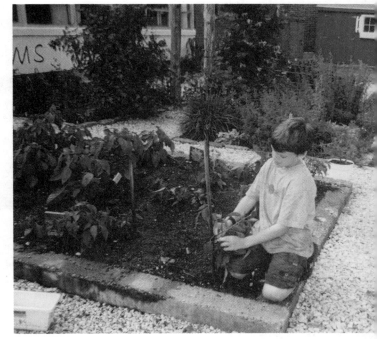

ALISA WRIGHT

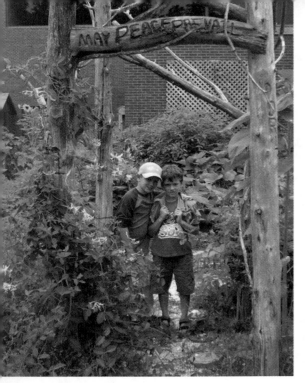

PHOTOS: ALISA WRIGHT

grade has a unique role: The kindergarten students make pickles and chutney from garden produce, first and third graders enter garden crops into fairs, and second- and fourth-grade students put the garden to bed once it's been picked clean. (Fifth graders prepare the beds for planting in the spring.)

Pizza-for-All Harvest Luncheon

When the sixth graders return in the fall, they immerse themselves in the garden, carefully observing, harvesting, and tasting the fruits of their labor. (They'll eventually return food scraps to the plots in the form of composted cafeteria waste.) Then they roll up their sleeves and prepare for the harvest luncheon.

"The class makes decisions about how to run the luncheon," says Alisa. (Cafeteria staff have already agreed to buy single-serving pizza shells.) "Just after Labor Day, students begin to prepare for the meal by harvesting, chopping, and dicing vegetables on tables in the classroom." Groups of students rotate through these prep stations. Some then sauté the produce in parent-donated skillets; others put together a garden-inspired salad or side dish such as tomato, basil, and onion salad; coleslaw; or roasted squash. A sign-up chart reveals who will do which jobs later that week: welcoming attendees, serving food, or conducting garden tours.

Donning the Harvest of Dreams aprons they have made (complete with a logo designed on a class computer), students serve up their fresh-flavored fare. The proud growers and chefs walk through the cafeteria offering samples of salads and pizza topping options. But it's not just the school community

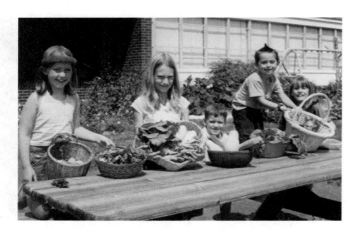

they nourish. "We invite lots of other people to the luncheon," explains Alisa. This includes a senior group, district administrators, members of the board of education, town officials, the Department of Environmental Protection's commissioner, uncles, parents, and others. "Students also give garden tours and talks about the history of the garden and how they plant and maintain it," says Alisa.

The Cooking Continues

The students' fun with cuisine doesn't stop there. Enthusiastic about preparing and relishing food together, the school community follows up with a vegetable-based cook-off. Each year features a specific item or flavorful theme such as eggplant, zucchini bread, or "a taste of tomatoes." "Each student brings in a favorite family recipe to share with classmates," explains Alisa. The group chooses one to make for the cook-off, and then divvies up the ingredient list.

On the appointed day, students pick and wash garden items. Schoolwide, sterilized classroom counters sport plug-in skillets, slow cookers, and bowls for batter (which is baked in school kitchen ovens). Each class prepares its recipe and sets the final, labeled product on a display table. Then in come the superintendent and other community members to judge the dishes on the basis of flavor, appearance, aroma, and texture. "Students eagerly await the results of the cook-off," says Alisa. "That's always a highlight." Then the feast begins.

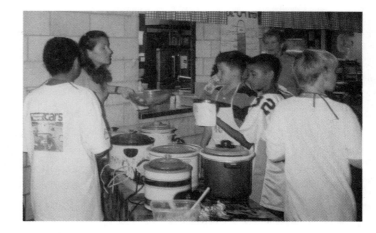

With so many years of tasty dishes under their belts, the young chefs would be remiss not to share the wealth. So the students, with guidance from the librarian, are authoring a cookbook to give to incoming families, sell to raise funds, or both.

How They Grow

Alisa and Paula agree that the Harvest of Dreams project has become a positive part of the school's culture. "Students who have been involved from year to year can hardly wait to be sixth graders," says Alisa. "After all, they are the key caretakers who everyone else looks up to. I've watched so many students shine in that role."

The project has surely met its main objective: Get students excited about tasting and trying new healthy foods. Student comments speak volumes about the impact of raising and tasting their own: "I never knew I liked beans or raw broccoli." Word has it that some students have led the way at home by introducing parents to new foods and flavors and to gardening. Then there are the personal and social benefits of producing something together that others value. "Their sense of working as a team is huge," says Alisa. "It's a real gift."

Testing and assessment are largely data driven, she explains. But the garden and cooking are connections with the real world that can involve the whole child. "They are nice diversions from all that 'mandated-ness' and there are countless opportunities for authentic learning." Take the compost project that school aide Zoë Greenwood moved forward. Student "compost cops" at each lunch session ensure that peers are properly saving leftovers. The kids can then see the results of this natural fertilizer on plants that, in turn, nourish the school community.

Students may not be the only ones influenced by the wonderful aromas emanating through the hallways each fall. The cafeteria manager has taken steps toward using more fresh vegetables in school meals.

One of their secrets: Cultivate enthusiasm for garden edibles in the cafeteria and classrooms!

Curriculum Serves Up Sensory Lessons

Food as Passport

Urban students learn about geography and cultures and open up to sampling new flavors with an award-winning exploratory food curriculum.

Hampstead Hill Academy
Baltimore, MD

Richard Daley Academy
Chicago, IL

When teachers at Hampstead Hill Academy in Baltimore, Maryland, retrieve their students from Ariel Demas' Food for Life class, they're met with an enthusiastic crowd eager to dish out nutritional and cultural facts, along with samples of the whole-food dishes they have just made. And that's no small thing. "One of my goals is to help dispel the perception that healthy food is scary and tastes weird," says Ariel. And she's not talking just about the students' responses.

Ariel's program, which was funded initially by the Food Studies Institute and local foundations, is based on a year-long, award-winning curriculum called *Food Is Elementary*. It features teaching tools, lessons, and recipes to help educators implement cooperative, multicultural cooking sessions. The curriculum engages all of a student's senses in learning about foods and nutrition. The kitchen equipment required is basic and can be used in any classroom — even those without sinks. (To learn more and order the *Food Is Elementary* curriculum, contact the Food Studies Institute: *www.foodstudies.org/Curriculum/*.)

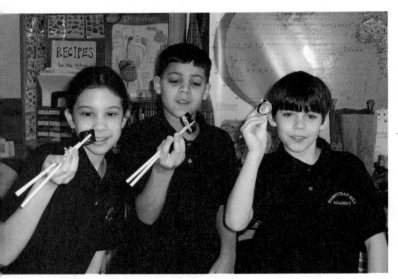

PHOTOS: ARIEL DEMAS/HAMPSTEAD HILL ACADEMY/FOOD STUDIES INSTITUTE

Kevin Read, a volunteer at Richard Daley Academy in Chicago, Illinois, used the same curriculum with a bilingual third-grade class. He admits that he was a bit of a skeptic at first. "I really had doubts," he says. "As good as the curriculum sounded, I assumed that kids, deep down, simply don't like vegetables." He soon changed his tune. Perhaps it was watching students devour raw Brussels sprouts! "When we explored edible plant part categories, we looked at those cool leaves wrapped up in tight balls," explains Kevin. That inspired students to want to taste them. "Most of the students are Mexican and had never seen them before, so they had no preconceptions," he adds. "Their first real hint was my comment that they might love them."

Laying the Groundwork: Digging into Edibles

The first half of the yearlong curriculum finds students handling and tasting fresh foods that represent different plant parts and food groups (e.g., grains, fruits), exploring the aesthetics of food, looking closely at product labels, and learning about what makes foods — and people — tick.

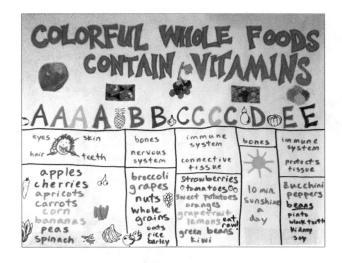

And sensory it is. A lesson on fat begins with students plunging their hands into butter. They learn that fat feels sticky, connect that to how it acts in our arteries, and then act like scientists as they "feel" milk samples and try to detect butterfat levels.

"Memorizing which vitamins do what doesn't make it," says Kevin. But keying into color codes does. He explains that one lesson helps students link different-colored foods to certain vitamins and general personal outcomes, such as good eyes or skin. Next, students list and draw foods representing each color; they add others throughout the year. Students in Ariel's classes even color-code their notes. The main message: Eat a rainbow of hues.

Another lesson invites students to examine, describe, taste, and write about different fruits, legumes, or whole-grain breads. But the youngsters' favorite might be the project for which they get to use food as an art medium! First they explore the colors and textures of different food items. As they cut and arrange them on white paper plates, whimsical creations emerge. Then the science slips in. Each artist must identify the vitamins in each item and its place on the food pyramid. Before eating their works, children draw or photograph them, admire one another's pieces, and explain what they were thinking as they designed their own.

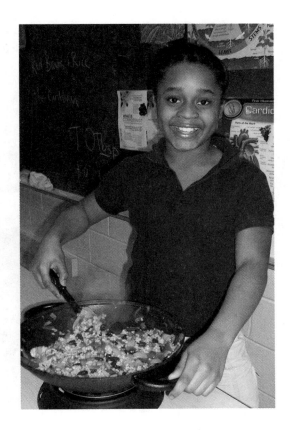

Cooking Across Cultures

Armed with a basic understanding and growing appreciation of food and nutrition, students spend the second semester cooking cuisines of other cultures. As they prepare each dish, they listen to music from the continent and learn something about the culture that created the recipe.

"The Indian dahl wasn't a huge favorite, but tabouli was," says Ariel. Red beans and rice also ranked high. Who would imagine that a tofu vegetable stir-fry would draw applause from kids? Using chopsticks was a real motivator for that meal, she explains.

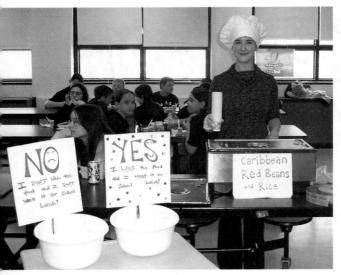

PHOTOS: ARIEL DEMAS/HAMPSTEAD HILL
ACADEMY/FOOD STUDIES INSTITUTE

Coaxing Converts

"No 'yuck' allowed" is one of the cardinal rules in Ariel's class. "I never pressure kids to try anything; but when the others do, they tend to get curious and step up." She also avoids pushing a heavy nutrition message, opting instead to engage students' hands and taste buds. "It's more important to get children thinking about what they're tasting and eating, where it comes from, and what they do and don't like," says Ariel.

It's not only the students who need enticing. Early on, Ariel invited the cafeteria staff to attend some Food for Life classes and try new dishes along with the kids. As they sampled the fare and encouraged students to keep open minds, the cooks and servers began to buy into the concept. Parents receive a newsletter filled with students' work, recipes, and comments about what they've been cooking. Some attend community dinners prepared by the school's culinary arts club. This year, parents and students can sign up to work together to prepare a weekly snack. (The recipe goes home with classmates.)

"Our principal is a great supporter," says Ariel. "He wants to see kids — and the staff — healthy and ready to learn." With that in mind, he first invited Ariel to cater all staff meetings so teachers could become more familiar with whole foods and model healthful eating for their students. Then after three successful years, he folded the program into the school budget. Next he helped Ariel pave the way for new dishes to someday land on the lunch counter. In 2007 she used new grant funds to conduct scientific food trials in the cafeteria. The goal: To offer tastes of popular dishes and determine which might pass muster with the student body. Using tickets to vote thumbs up or down, a majority of students opted for burritos, red beans and rice, North African stew, and others from the Food is Elementary curriculum.

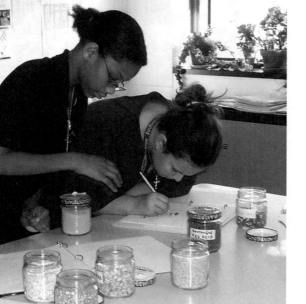

How They Grow

"Beyond getting an introduction to new foods and cooking techniques, students gain a new way of looking at food: how it connects to cultures, its beauty, and the fun we can have preparing it," says Kevin. He adds that as food themes are integrated into other subjects, the students see how their learning relates to real life.

Perhaps less tangible are the benefits that accrue when students are treated as responsible, able learners. For example, they use adult-size knives to cut vegetables — but not without some instruction. Even before students hold a knife, Kevin asks them to draw and label one (blade, handle, sharp and dull sides). Then he shows them how to hold the knife and food (with a "claw grip" to keep the joints vertical). "The students appreciate that they are trusted to use a serious and powerful tool that I tell them will enable them to eat good foods," explains Kevin.

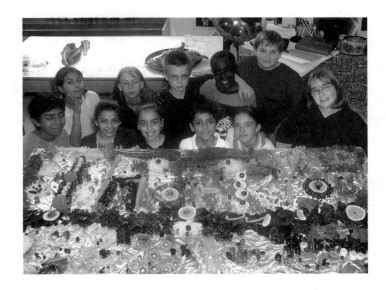

"The world of food is opening up for these children, most of whom are from very poor families," says Ariel. "Because it's so sensory-based, the kids remember what they've explored and eaten. In fact, I hear stories from parents whose youngsters have requested foods we've tasted." At least one of her students reported that his family switched from white to whole-grain bread.

But she admits that it's not always a quick turnaround. "The kids may read labels now and get grossed out by the ingredients, but still choose to buy the items." The lesson on fats, she adds, hasn't precluded youngsters from wanting food from McDonald's. But little changes are apparent, and they're beginning to influence family behavior.

> "One of my goals is to help dispel the perception that healthy food is scary and tastes weird."
> — Ariel Demas, Hampstead Hill Academy

Nourishing School Fundraiser

Farm Foods, Friendships, Finances Flourish

During farm visits, students learn how local agriculture improves the stability and health of their community. With help from the Natural Resources Conservation Service, they peddle farm goods in a win-win business venture.

**Central Lake Elementary
Central Lake, MI**

If an eyebrow was raised when Jeff Kessler's fourth graders revealed the price of the jam they were peddling, the students had a ready response. After all, they'd seen just how long it took to pick and process the raspberries. They would sweeten the "sell" by explaining to potential customers that farmers like Tom Cooper were their neighbors who grew or made products by hand — not in a factory.

Homegrown fundraising in Central Lake, Michigan, was the innovation of school parent Pepper Bromelmeier. She had once received a survey asking how she liked the school's annual candy sale. Her response: Not at all. "But I didn't want to just write back without offering some sort of alternative idea," says Pepper. Her work with farmers through the federal Natural Resources Conservation Service provided the spark — and a winning solution. She knew that many area family farmers, squeezed by low bulk commodity prices, were creating specialty products and seeking local markets. "I wondered if farmers I knew might be interested in selling products for a school fundraising project, so I made some calls," explains Pepper. All were eager to participate.

Once the PTO realized that Pepper's proposed Farmer to Community Connection project was manageable, they signed on, too. After all, it also had the potential to link students to healthful fresh foods; teach them about the local food system; and give them a practical context for learning and applying skills in math, language arts, and beyond.

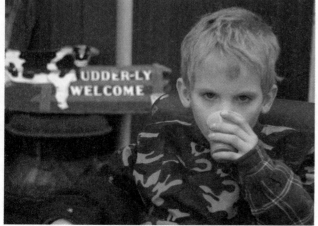

Farm Visits Set the Stage

The farmers' product suggestions yielded a palette of healthful (and healthfully produced) items: apples, dried cherries, fruit salsa, squash, honey, pasture-raised bison, goat's-milk soap, trout, chickens, and more. Before any transactions occurred, Jeff's young entrepreneurs paid a visit to four of the 12 farms whose products they would promote.

"The kids were connected to this fundraiser much more than to others we've done," says Jeff. "They had a personal stake because they knew for whom they were selling the products and why these neighbors were passionate about their work." Pepper greased the wheels by suggesting that each farmer introduce a concept that would help show the importance of the business to the economy and community. For instance, one woman had a flow chart with "smiley" faces representing people who work on her farm. She explained how the farm income also supported the jobs of other people — and businesses — in the community. (Community is an important topic of study in the fourth-grade curriculum.)

During the field trips, Jeff also asked farmers to high-light aspects of their products that students could use to pitch them. For instance, a dairy farmer revealed that his cows listened to classical music and that peaceful cows gave better milk. And imagine the creative images for marketing posters inspired by a farmer contributing pasture-raised poultry who plucked a chicken out of the freezer and said, "This chicken is as big as my head!"

On-site lessons in business and farm economics opened students' eyes, but the samples of items such as "natural" chocolate milk, cherries, and bison burger bites made the experience worth writing home about.

Enterprising Lessons

"We always used the term 'business partners' when we shook hands with the food producers," says Jeff. As the youngsters worked through the logistics and economics, and pitched products in person and via letters, their budding business became a laboratory for lessons in several subject areas. For instance, they set prices for products after looking at what stores charged and discussing cost considerations with farmers.

"At first, students thought it was unfair to sell something for more than they'd paid the farmer for the product," says Jeff. But as they calculated how much they'd earn if they made X amount per item and sold Y items, students learned about profits and changed their tune! "Our profit margin (around 30 percent) was much greater than students had earned selling trinkets from overseas," explains Jeff. (These days, the school's 30 fourth graders sell about $4,000 worth of products in two weeks and net $1,400 in profit.) Harder to measure are the rewards students reaped as they built bridges to the local farm community and began to grasp how food, communities, and health are intertwined.

FARM FUNDRAISING PROJECT TIMELINE

Early to Mid-Fall: Students, teachers, and parent volunteers visit farms.

After the Farm Tours:

❀ Students create posters, brochures, and other marketing materials. They also display samples of nonperishable items in a hallway showcase. (If possible, set this up before parent/teacher conferences.)

❀ Organizer creates order forms and a sheet describing each farm and its products, its location, and where and when it sells products. Some go home with students; others are posted in community locations.

❀ During the two weeks of sales, teachers conduct standards-based classroom lessons that relate to the fundraiser.

❀ Students or staff add up quantities of items on order forms, come up with a total for each item for each producer, and contact farmers.

❀ Teachers and parent volunteers pick up items at farms about one or two weeks after the preset selling time. (Perishable items are put in school fridge.)

❀ Parent volunteers pack items into individual orders. Customers come in during set pickup times. (Customers usually like having items ready just prior to Thanksgiving.)

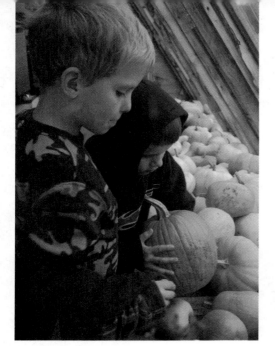

PHOTOS: TOM BROWN/NORTHERN
EXPOSURES PHOTOGRAPHY

Meanwhile, producers involved in the project have appreciated having a new source of free advertising. Their revenues aren't enough to make a big dent in the local farm economy — at least not yet. But when the director of Michigan's Department of Agriculture learned about the program, he vowed to help agriculture and education officials consider whether they could help spread the program to schools across the state.

Advice on Farm Fundraisers

First, suggest Pepper and Jeff, line up a small group of farmers and other product suppliers. Meet with them and make sure that they are comfortable addressing kids and understand the spirit of the project. Then approach the school board, if necessary.

If you don't have connections with local farmers, contact your county Natural Resources Conservation Service office for help. You'll find links to state offices here: *www.nrcs.usda.gov/about/organization/regions.html*. You can also try your local university Cooperative Extension office and nonprofit groups that promote local farm foods.

Make sure to sign up parents and other volunteers to help break down piles of food and other products into individual orders; if you don't, you'll have a bottleneck.

Start with interested teachers, and let the program's success entice others to participate. "Once teachers saw the farm fundraiser work well, they got it and became great supporters," says Pepper.

It... had the potential to link students to healthful fresh foods; teach them about the local food system; and give them a practical context for learning and applying skills in math, language arts, and beyond.

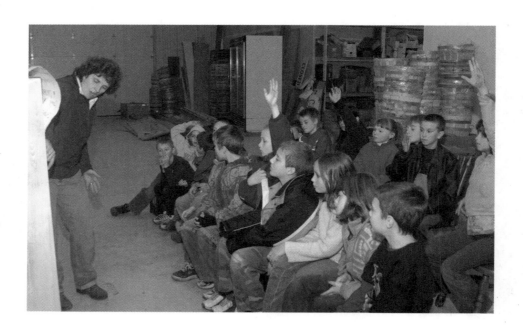

Homegrown Lunch

"Trying to get the foodservice to incorporate new and healthier foods can be daunting — especially in a big district like ours," says Clare Seguin, elementary science teacher at Lincoln School in Madison, Wisconsin. "They seem to think they have to somehow trick students into eating vegetables. But people underestimate kids' culinary savvy." She contends that when vegetables are really fresh, kids love them, and that it's worth pushing the envelope. And Clare would know. It's hard not to notice when your students devour raw daikon radishes and sweet potatoes!

Clare's school is a pilot site in the Wisconsin Homegrown Lunch (WHL) program. Started in 2001 by a parent, WHL is now a collaboration between a local-foods group (Research, Education, Action, and Policy on Food Group) and the University of Wisconsin Center for Integrated Agricultural Systems. Its goal is to link classrooms and school cafeterias with nearby farms and restaurants. This translates into opportunities for students to learn about the local food system and nutrition, and opportunities to create new markets for farmers.

Simple Farm Snacks

One of the initial projects "seemed too simple and obvious," says Project Coordinator Doug Wubben. Once a week, all classrooms in one school would get locally grown carrots for snack. Still, it took some finagling to make it happen because lunchroom staff didn't have time to prepare the snacks. So a local food coop offered to cut and bag carrot "coins" for 20 classes, and a teacher agreed to pick them up. Says Clare, "The kids loved it and never seemed to get tired of them." But Doug set his sights on getting a different snack each week and involving more schools. Now, farmers deliver organic cherry tomatoes, peppers, sweet potatoes, and more to the district foodservice or to the coop for preparation. Once a week the items go out with the regular foodservice deliveries to four schools. Educators receive a newsletter called Snack Bites that highlights the featured snack and the farm it came from along with related activities and lessons.

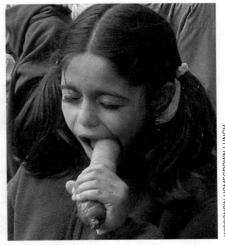

WISCONSIN HOMEGROWN LUNCH

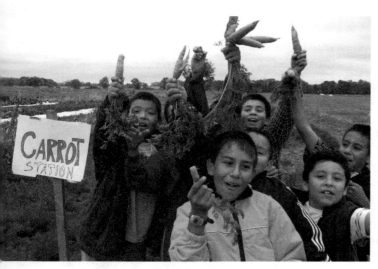

PHOTOS: WISCONSIN HOMEGROWN LUNCH

The snack food costs are covered by a small grant and PTA funds, but Doug continues to look for ways to keep the farm-fresh snacks coming. This includes asking parents to contribute a small amount of money in lieu of sending in their own snacks. (The PTA could help cover the cost for low-income families).

Local Farms Rule

"Our fourth graders have the dairy message reinforced often, but they should also know that local farms produce much more," says Doug. To that end, he has worked with farmers to develop on-farm activity stations that engage visiting students. Clare's class rotated through a series of such stations. They shucked beans, separated and planted garlic, spread cover crop seeds, dug and tasted carrots, and "fed" compost piles. They even went to the spring, where the farmer talked about preserving safe groundwater by using organic growing techniques. "One time, we actually prepared lunch using foods that had been raised on the farm," says Clare. "Those experiences really stuck with the kids."

> "*When vegetables are really fresh, kids love them, and… it's worth pushing the envelope.*"
> — Clare Seguin, science teacher, Lincoln School, Madison, Wisconsin

Classroom Activities Reinforce Local Food Mantra

Some Wisconsin farmers also go into the schools and work with students on simple interactive activities they developed. One memory game uses a set of cards for each season that depicts vegetables kids can eat at that time. A "harvest vegetable" activity invites students to observe and feel cards with real vegetable seeds and images of the full-grown produce. "Someone always wonders why one of the cards has chunks of potatoes in place of seeds," says Doug.

Clare's students took on related activities: tasting and comparing heirloom tomatoes or different apple varieties, and making vegetable wraps in preparation for a pilot "homegrown lunch." Every spring, each student gets a cherry tomato seedling to nurture. He or she works to keep it thriving at home over the summer and returns in the fall "with great stories and bowls full of cherry tomatoes to share," says Clare.

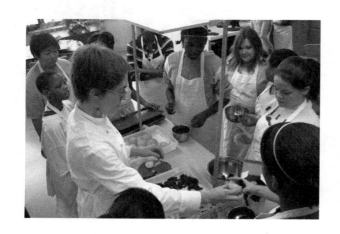

After each classroom activity, a letter goes home with students explaining what they did in class. Accompanying worksheets get parents and kids working together as scientists; they might compare food tastes, textures, and other qualities. When they reach middle school, some students in the district get to dig even deeper by opting for a "healthy snacking" class or chef-in-the-classroom program.

Farm to Cafeteria: Tackling Challenges

Doug and his colleagues have encountered plenty of bumps along the way as they've tried to bring their vision to reality. Important steps in the process, he advises, are building relationships and understanding what barriers exist. "Initially, we sat down with school foodservice people in the district and shared some of the current statistics on childhood nutrition and obesity," says Doug. "We explained that we're aware of the issues and have explored successes of other farm to school programs. Then we shared some of the kinds of things we'd like to get going."

He describes one of the biggest hurdles his group is working to overcome: "Our school district has a central kitchen that prepares and packs up to 15,000 meals a day for 47 schools. And they don't have time for a lot of food preparation." With that in mind, he's sought ways to get local food to the kitchen in forms that are easier to use. The food coop partnership has been the most fruitful one. When the foodservice agreed to test some new menu items, such as chili and sweet potato/carrot muffins, the coop kitchen shredded, cut, and mashed the vegetables. Doug "brokered" that venture, but the foodservice and coop now negotiate directly with each other.

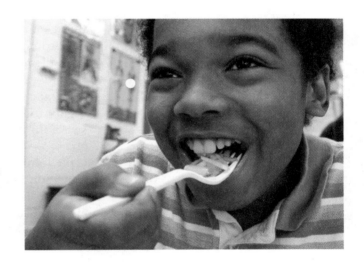

"We need to feed kids' bodies well in order to effectively feed their minds," says Doug. "Schools are well aware of this, as evidenced by the healthy snacks offered to students on testing days. Everyone's aware of the problem, and solutions exist; our job is to help create the local and political will to work on making changes."

Locally Flavored Fundraisers

According to Doug, it's important to work on more than one school food front. After all, the lunchroom is just one of the places where children and food meet. To that end, he joined with a parent group to offer a fresh take on an entrenched ritual: school fundraisers. "Our 'homegrown holiday' fundraiser was a refreshing alternative to those that are outlets for unhealthy foods and other items parents feel pressured to buy." The gift items included a winter vegetable box; a "bee box" featuring honey, candles, and honey sticks; cheeses; chocolate-covered cranberries; dried cherries; popcorn; and other products from local farms and businesses. After paying wholesale prices to the farmers and craftspeople, the school cleared a whopping $2,400 from this pre-holiday sale. Other schools in the system have followed suit, investing part of the proceeds in farm to school projects.

To learn more about Wisconsin Homegrown Lunch, visit: *www.reapfoodgroup.org/farmtoschool/*.

> "We need to feed kids' bodies well in order to effectively feed their minds."
>
> — Doug Wubben, Project Coordinator

Savoring Flavors
in Las Cruces

A Tasting Program Delivers

A dietitian finds funding, along with support from school- and district-level foodservice staff, to buy, deliver, and prepare produce for a tasting curriculum.

Las Cruces Public Schools
Las Cruces, NM

"I don't think anyone gets much out of teaching the facts about nutrients," says Barbara Berger, dietitian for the Las Cruces, New Mexico, public schools. She notes that even the food pyramid can be dry if it's taught out of context. But it's a different tale altogether when students have repeated opportunities to observe and draw new fruits and vegetables, taste them, use colorful language to describe their flavors, vote for those that spark their taste buds, and explore each item's cultural connections. Intrigued by that image, Barbara created a pilot food-tasting program, which she patterned after the successful Cooking with Kids project (see page 61).

She knew that the local university was the subcontractor for the federal Food Stamp Nutrition Education (FSNE) program. (The program allocates funds for use in schools that have more than 50 percent of students on free or reduced lunches.) Because many schools in Barbara's large urban district fit the bill, she proposed a pilot tasting project. Her entry point: school nurses. "The nurses loved the concept, saw it as a strategy for obesity prevention, and went back and sold the idea to the principals," she explains. But it's the support of the district's foodservice that made the program logistics palatable.

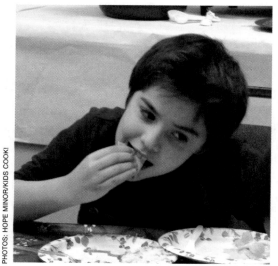

PHOTOS: HOPE MINOR/KIDS COOK!

The Logistics: Getting Food to Schools

Before students could try even a morsel, Barbara needed a plan for obtaining produce and delivering it to the nine participating schools. "The district foodservice has storage facilities, delivery schedules, and buying power," reasoned Barbara. It helped that the department employed her and that its staff had already begun to delve into nutrition education. Today, its buyers purchase what she needs for tasting sessions, and they deliver it to each school. In the interest of efficiency, each classroom in the district gets the same goods on the same day.

Barbara manages to get some local items, but points out that it takes time to build relationships with growers and find large quantities of certain foods. Pecans and pistachios from an area farmer were a no-brainer, but her dream of having local fresh peas for a tasting session had to be postponed. "The local farms couldn't grow nearly enough for me, but my plan for next year is to contact larger farmers who have an interest in schools and agricultural education," says Barbara. "If local growers were able to ramp up to meet our demands, we could have a significant impact on the agricultural economy."

Grant money covers the raw goods and pays for school foodservice workers to prepare tasting "kits" for each classroom. Before each new session, Barbara e-mails the staffs, introducing the theme of that month's kit and explaining how to prepare it: cleaning, cutting or scoring, weighing, bagging, and so on. Some kits include classroom equipment (e.g., apple corers), purchased at discounts through the foodservice's vendors. The district print shop makes enough copies of student materials for each classroom.

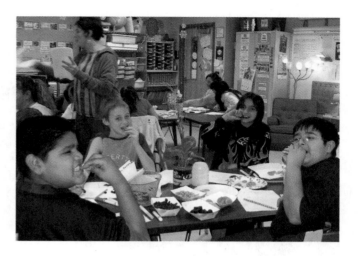

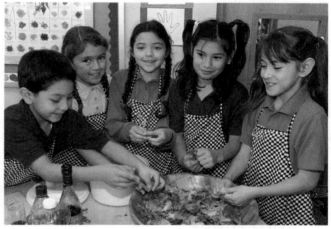

LYNN WALTERS, COOKING WITH KIDS, INC.

Cultivating Curious Palates

Before they feed students fresh fare, teachers are lured to attend an hour-long inservice workshop by the promise of free nutrition education materials. There, Barbara models a tasting lesson and engages teachers as learners.

Come monthly tasting days, each teacher sends a student to the cafeteria at a set time to pick up a classroom kit. "For the introductory tastings, participants can choose anything they want," says Barbara. She's managed to score items such as prickly pear cactus leaves (for a New Mexico theme), avocados, and plums. For the remainder of the sessions, Barbara preselects foods such as apples; dried fruits, nuts, and seeds; citrus fruits; salads; grapes; peas; and sunflower sprouts. Coordinating the timing of certain fresh items with the school calendar is a bit tricky, but melons and tomatoes might be in the mix!

Reflecting the district's commitment to language acquisition through the strategy of "total physical response," students employ descriptive language as they observe, taste, discuss, and write about the day's edible. They also learn a bit about its history, its cultural connections, and, yes, even its nutritional value.

As they repeat the process with each new edible, students begin to shed their assumptions about what foods they dislike, becoming more willing to take

Look within the school system to see how the work might be shared and divided.
— Barbara Berger, public schools dietitian, Las Cruces, New Mexico

risks and try new things. In the end, says Barbara, students come to see food in a different way and discover that healthful eats can make awesome nacks.

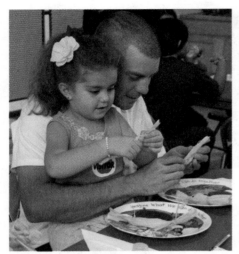

LYNN WALTERS, COOKING WITH KIDS, INC.

Nurturing Home Connections

When families come to school for parent nights, they get to sample similar fare at Barbara's fruit and vegetable exhibit. After deciding which items they prefer, parents and their young charges register their opinions on a master bar graph. Barbara explains that one parent finally "got" her child's new passion for kiwi as she dabbled with new flavors herself.

"We don't ram nutrients down anybody's throat," explains Barbara. "We assume most people already know that fruits and vegetables are healthy." But she does make interactive parent/child homework sheets that extend classroom experiences. For example, a treasure hunt sheet asks the parent and child to go to the store and pick out a new fruit or vegetable they haven't tried before. "Next, they draw, taste, and describe it, and circle happy faces to show their preferences for the item," says Barbara. The final directive: Interview another family member, register his or her preference, and compare the data. At least one parent thinks the strategy works: "I strongly feel that the students are educating [us] in many cases where parents haven't purchased the fruits or vegetables because they've never tasted them."

> *If local growers were able to ramp up to meet our demands, we could have a significant impact on the agricultural economy.*
>
> — Barbara Berger,
> public schools dietitian,
> Las Cruces, New Mexico

Advice on Getting Started

Start small, Barbara suggests. "Don't take on as much as I did." She notes that the Cooking with Kids program cofounders started with just two schools that had supportive staffs and principals. Then find partners. "Look within the school system to see how the work might be shared and divided. Don't forget that school nurses — and of course, the foodservice — can be great allies." Finally, identify funding. Running a tasting program like this can get pricey. "Find out which agency or agencies in your state manage the funds for the federal Food Stamp Nutrition Education (FSNE) program and propose an idea," says Barbara. (Start with your state universities and Cooperative Extension offices.) Recipients need to match the food stamp funds. Barbara's solution: Have everyone involved with the project keep records of time spent; those hours can be part of the match. For a list of state contacts for the FSNE program, visit: *www.csrees.usda.gov/nea/food/fsne/progmap_text.cfm.*

Cooking with Kids Program: Cuisine, Cultures, Curriculum

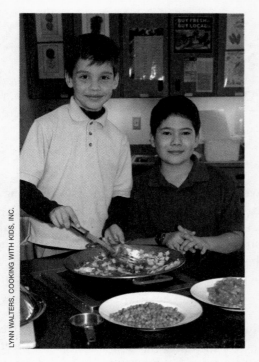

LYNN WALTERS, COOKING WITH KIDS, INC.

Kids are five to 20 times as likely to eat a food again if they've had a hand in preparing it, says Cornell University researcher Antonia Demas. That concept, and a desire to improve school food, inspired parent and chef Lynn Walters to initiate a hands-on food and nutrition program in two Santa Fe, New Mexico, public schools in 1995. The upshot was the Cooking with Kids integrated curriculum for grades K–6. The 11-session program engages students in tasting fresh fruits and vegetables, using them to cook dishes from diverse cultures, and exploring their travels and life stories.

Lynn and program director Jane Stacey have since published the curriculum and expanded the program to 11 schools. About twice a month, every public school in the city also features a Cooking with Kids lunch. Through the state's farm to school program, participating schools can obtain edibles with local roots. The program's successful model and materials have sparked offshoots in other regions. The Savoring Flavors and Appetizing Lessons profiles highlight how two groups of educators modified the successful Cooking with Kids concept to meet local needs.

On the project's Web site (*www.cookingwithkids.net*), you can learn more about the origins and details of Cooking with Kids, download free tasting lessons, and order bilingual (Spanish/English) cooking and tasting curricula, a DVD, and school lunch recipes.

Appetizing Lessons in "Kids Cook!" Classrooms

"Kids who have opportunities to taste foods are willing to accept more variety," says Hope Miner, founding director of a nonprofit called Kids Cook. But the real meat, in her book, is in the experience of cooking. It's not just the flavors that are worth savoring, but their fusion with cultural connections and curriculum that makes her Kids Cook program such a winner.

Inspired by the Cooking with Kids founders and curriculum (see page 61), Hope has tailored her program and materials to meet the unique needs of her locality (Albuquerque, New Mexico) and large urban school district.

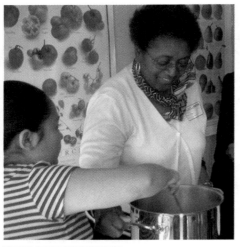

PHOTOS: HOPE MINOR/KIDS COOK!

Studying Cultural Cuisine and Customs

"We first came up with a curriculum that focused on five regions of the U.S.," says Hope. The regional themes reflect the country's history and its melting pot of cultures. For instance, a traditional African-American black-eyed pea and rice dish (hoppin' John), accompanied by cooked fresh greens, was the entrée for flavors and stories of the south. "Yes, kids eat and love greens!" says Hope.

Today the program features five cooking units from the United States and an eight-unit global collection of dishes and lessons. Students not only get to cut carrots and sample fresh ginger for the Chinese soup, but use chopsticks, learn a few new words in a foreign tongue, and make noodles from scratch. The colorful history of potatoes comes to life as young chefs create potato dishes for a Peruvian meal and discover that the natives use a different type of spud for each of a dozen different dishes. Geography can be a bore. But when students take out maps to identify the origins of ingredients and dishes they've made, they develop an appetite for learning.

How It Works

Like Barbara Berger, Hope receives funding through the university-administered Food Stamp Nutrition Education (FSNE) program for eligible schools.

Additional support from General Mills enables the program to extend into non-qualifying schools.

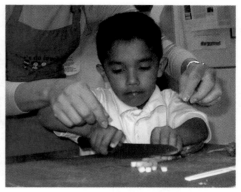

It can be awkward if alluring aromas waft from only some classrooms in the building, so when Kids Cook agrees to take on a school, every child is involved. Each youngster in the nine participating schools receives 13 hours of tasting, cooking, sanitation, and food safety classes during the year. All schools implement the same unit at once, which simplifies purchasing and scheduling.

Before students dig in, teachers must come to a two-hour Cooking with Teachers training to learn about program expectations. For instance, the school must provide a dedicated refrigerator and paper towels, and make extra copies of materials. The program covers everything else. A Kids Cook staff person — professional nutritionist, educator, or someone who simply loves food and children — rolls in a cooking cart with burners, a griddle, food preparation tools, and ingredients. For their Southwestern regional meal, kids in Albuquerque turn out homemade whole-wheat flour tortillas, blue corn pancakes, black bean salad, and calabacitas (a summer squash dish).

"We break down each recipe to feed four to eight people," says Hope. This means that after donning chefs' hats in school, youngsters can share their culinary skills with families. Once a month, the central kitchen also makes a Kids Cook recipe adapted for large quantities and distributes the meal to all 93 elementary schools in the district. This has sparked tremendous interest in duplicating the program and has enticed more parents, alert to the quality of the meals, to join their youngsters in the cafeteria on Kids Cook days.

Advice on Engaging Students

"In 25 years of teaching, I've never heard a parent say, 'Johnny's excited that you're teaching the food guide pyramid,'" says Hope. "Nutrition education must engage students, include healthy foods, and teach about variety and moderation." She explains that as the Kids Cook staff teaches students to prepare foods they love, they discuss where key ingredients fit on the food pyramid and how the main nutrients keep kids healthy. "Students may talk about iron in the context of the food they just ate, but you can't lecture them into learning that," says Hope. She also advises flexibility, noting that you'll need to adjust and meet the needs of the populations with whom you work.

Finally, says Hope, "Go where your heart is. We started this project with no money and two really committed people wanting to make a difference." And so they did — if demand is any indicator. The Kids Cook five-year waiting list features every school in the district! Ineligible schools have even solicited outside grants and offered to pay their own way.

Take Action

STARTING A PROGRAM

Hope is committed to getting this type of nutrition education out to as many people as possible. To that end, she is delighted to help others plan and execute programs. You can contact her via the Kids Cook Web site (*www.kidscook.us*).

Good Things Cooking
in North Carolina

Farmers and Chefs Help Young Minds Grow

Students' enthusiasm for school garden produce inspires parents and an agricultural nonprofit to improve district cafeteria offerings through food education. Kids and foodservice staff connect with and learn from farmers and local chefs.

Ashville City Schools
Buncombe County Schools, NC

"I didn't start out to create a farm to school project," says educator Emily Jackson from Asheville, North Carolina. It began with a school garden. "I saw how much our garden entranced my third graders. And when they grew the food, they always wanted to eat it." What's more, they paid full attention to related lessons in Emily's classroom. Knowing she was on to something, Emily got other teachers involved. But, she says, something was missing. "We were growing good food, but we weren't connecting it to the cafeteria."

Emily's goal was modest: To grow a new generation of people who cared where their food came from! To that end, she worked with the Appalachian Sustainable Agriculture Project and secured a grant for a project dubbed Growing Minds. Soon the gardens became part of a broader nutrition and farm to school program that now includes farm visits, classroom cooking, chef demos, and cafeteria connections.

"Too often, nutrition education is uninteresting, lots of facts are delivered, and the focus is on what kids shouldn't be doing," says Emily. Her philosophy? Find out what engages students. What do they know about foods and what would they like to know? Help teachers think about their current instructional goals and plans, and ask, "How do garden, food, farm, and cooking connections fit in?"

Cooking Classes Flourish

A concerned parent group called Eat Better, Learn Better discussed how to engage students with good foods rather than lecture them about bad ones. In-school cooking sessions seemed like a good springboard. In participating schools, a volunteer cook came in once a week or so. He or she (usually a parent, chef, or nutritionist) brought in a seasonal recipe, ingredients, and related local products. Teachers could sign up to send 10 students to a class. Recipes always went home in Spanish and English.

"One chef heard that the kids liked tasting kohlrabi, so she proposed a carrot/kohlrabi stew," says Emily. The meal was a hit even with young skeptics — as was the guacamole and the winter squash/apple dish. Another chef

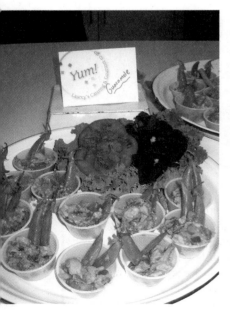

APPALACHIAN SUSTAINABLE AGRICULTURE PROJECT

pushed the envelope by suggesting chicken mafe, an African chicken, peanut butter, cabbage, and carrot dish. It, too, got a thumbs-up from the kids. As students' skills grew, so did their culinary wisdom. One boy observed, "Things taste better when you add the right stuff to them." Word has it that many students have also influenced their parents' food choices.

Training Chefs to Mentor Students

Emily was concerned about "burning out" the few volunteer chefs. When she and colleagues solicited others who might like to work with children, they got an overwhelming response. A local foundation grant enabled her group to train the food experts to work with students and support the school curriculum. During the first hour of the "Chef Fest" session, the facilitators discussed which curriculum concepts for each grade could easily tie in with cooking. They also shared some basic advice with the chefs: Use simple ingredients; be aware of local cultural influences on children's food experiences; bring in related kids' fiction; and so on. A chef who had already worked with students came to discuss his experiences and how the restaurant benefited from the exposure. After that, the real fun began.

"We set up four stations with portable propane burners and we posted the curriculum connections on the wall," says Emily. The chefs had brought in ingredients. (She suggests having students bring in some items or purchasing them with grant funds.) Third and fourth graders worked with the chefs to create and consume an apple and winter squash soup. If it hadn't rained, says Emily, the cooking sessions would have occurred in the school garden so students could educate chefs about what grows there. "After the kids left, we spent a couple of hours discussing the experience." Then the kid-savvy chefs repeated the cooking session with students in grades K–2; they again debriefed as a group. Participants left with a notebook of lesson plans written by a teacher Emily had hired.

Today, when a teacher or school wants to set up a chef connection, someone contacts Emily's program. Growing Minds maintains a database of chefs interested in working with schools and the age groups and numbers of students they're willing to take on. At least one chef also does a monthly cooking demonstration for school kitchen workers, discussing cooking strategies and ingredients, and fielding questions.

Fifth-grade teacher Janet Miller says that her students have been delighted by the generosity of the chefs, one of whom donated a set of aprons for students to don as they cook. "They've also become much more willing to try different things and do the work involved in growing ingredients." She believes that such firsthand experiences with people who are passionate

Fresh Idea

TIP: FARMERS' MARKET SCAVENGER HUNT

"I designed a scavenger hunt sheet for a farmers' market visit," says Emily. Her goal was to pique students' interest and focus them on some science concepts. But something more personal happened, too. With scavenger hunt sheets in hand, the young sleuths were more apt to talk with the men and women who grew their food. Student questions often broke the ice: "Some students, challenged to find something that grows underground, ran up to a farmer to ask if his lettuce would fit the bill!" says Emily.

> "We make sure the foodservice staff knows they are an important part of these efforts."
> — Emily Jackson, Growing Minds

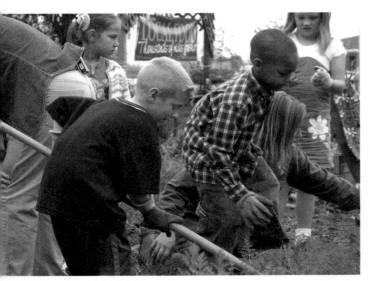

PHOTOS: APPALACHIAN SUSTAINABLE
AGRICULTURE PROJECT

about cooking and sharing good meals help pave the way for healthy lifelong relationships with food.

From Farm to Restaurant

When a K–2 class visited a local farm, parents weren't the only escorts. A local chef joined the group to help students focus on the foods they were seeing. The plan: Invite the class back to the restaurant the following day. "The chef had noticed how excited the kids were when they saw and tasted beautiful okra at the farm," says Emily. "So she talked about things they might do with it back at the restaurant." The next day, she prepared some okra in different ways (such as pickled, and fried with cornmeal) for the class to taste and describe. A stunned and grateful parent sent this note to the chef: "When we went to the grocery store, my child begged me to buy okra and insisted that we try cooking it three different ways. Thank you!"

During the farm visit and restaurant session, one of the adults captured youngsters' comments and "incredible conversations" on tape. After a volunteer edited and narrated the tape, it ran on a local radio station, garnering great public relations for the project. It should also prove valuable for soliciting donations from potential funders.

Fresh from a year of new flavors and farm connections, a group of K–2 students worked with Emily and another teacher to create a book about their experiences. Language arts lessons bloomed as students determined what type of book it would be ("nonfiction, because this is real") and what audience they would target ("other kids like us"). The storyline: Who grows our food and the experiences we had cooking it. The group incorporated photos, students' drawings, and quotes they'd pulled from field trip audiotapes. Money from the project's grant covered printing costs.

Growing Ties with the Cafeteria

Early on in the project, in an effort to better understand how the foodservice operated, Emily spent a day shadowing the child nutrition director, the person in charge of all food for the school system. "I hadn't realized that the school food budget was totally separate from the rest of the school," says Emily. "Or that the foodservice has to raise all its own money."

So she spread the word, first to the Eat Better, Learn Better group. The upshot: The group asked the foodservice for a cafeteria "wish list." Then they sent the list home with students; families who could do so bought list items from a restaurant supplier. The parent group also bought a share in a community supported agriculture (CSA) farm so they could have fresh produce for cooking classes and cafeteria demos without taxing the foodservice budget. As the farm to school program grew, Emily used a grant from a

> **If kids had this experience, we would have no problem getting them to eat veggies.**
> — Urban Food Worker

local health and wellness trust fund to buy "personal" CSA shares to get foodservice managers excited about fresh foods.

Meanwhile, Emily worked on a broader scale by starting a district-wide farm to school committee made up of child nutrition directors, farmers, Cooperative Extension staff, the health department, and a local food-processing facility. Committee members suspected that some food workers might be hesitant to support the project, so they took them on field trips to meet the growers and see what they had to offer. "These urban cooks tasted fresh corn and ate their way across the farm," says Emily. Said one, "If kids had this experience, we would have no problem getting them to eat veggies." During the locally grown picnic lunch, the school cooks got to discuss their experiences and concerns with growers.

"We make sure the foodservice staff knows they are an important part of these efforts," says Emily. And, it appears, they're rising to the challenge. Now, posters featuring photos of a supplier's farm are prominently displayed in the lunchroom. As students enter, they can read the companion stories of the family and farm behind the fresh wholesome fare. At one school, a meet-the-farmer event included a stir-fry cooking demo along with samples. "The foodservice manager hadn't had much success peddling cooked cabbage," says Emily. But when she replicated what the farmer had done, it was wildly successful!

Find a Farm Field Trip Tool Kit, recipes, and more information about Growing Minds on the program's Web site: *www.growing-minds.org/*.

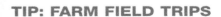
Fresh Idea

TIP: FARM FIELD TRIPS

"Field trips can directly and indirectly enhance a farmer's income," says Emily. But, she adds, many farmers are scared to death about what to do with a group of kids. So why not pay them to get together with the experts? Growing Minds set up a workshop for farmers and teachers. Each group got to talk about what it needed from the other ("Bathrooms," said one teacher), and presenters from both audiences described how they'd made the visits enriching for kids.

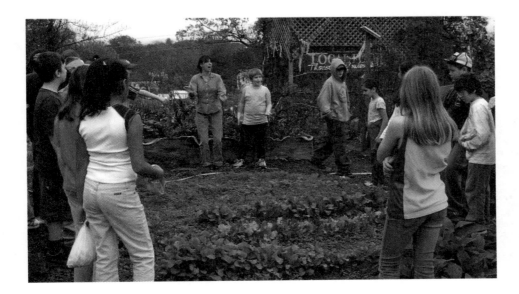

Local Foods Rule

It was the cheese topping. Something was terribly wrong. Traverse City, Michigan, principal Sharon Dionne couldn't find a shred of real cheese on the ingredient list. That's when she and a handful of concerned parents and teachers set up the Nutrition Advisory Council. Four years later, lunch-line cheese is the real thing, white bread is but a memory, and students raise food in a "kid-driven" edible garden. What's more, they learn loads from local farmers whose fresh fare — and tales — they relish. And that's just the beginning.

Launching a Nutrition Council

"Our Nutrition Advisory Council began as a subcommittee of our regular Parent Teacher Organization (PTO)," says council cofounder and parent Dana Goodwin. She explains that the idea of spearheading change in an institutional setting seemed daunting at first. So the group did its homework, researching successful nutrition initiatives across the country and drawing from the best of them. It surveyed families to determine whether the availability of more fresh locally grown produce would spur them to participate in the school's lunch program. (The answer was yes.) Then members hammered out a mission and goals with an eye toward long-term systemic change.

At first the group met monthly. "But finding times that would work for at-home parents, teachers, and community members was a challenge," says Dana. Now the group gets together less frequently, but between gatherings they share information and updates via e-mail. In preparation for a planning session, members might read an online article that gets them thinking about issues and possibilities. The Center for Ecoliteracy's *Thinking Outside the Lunchbox* essays offer great food for thought, says Dana.

Council members were encouraged to visit the school cafeteria before meetings and perhaps load a plate with fresh salad fixings or sample a new local item. "What better way to monitor and measure our progress?" asks Dana. "This past spring, we were delighted to see fresh

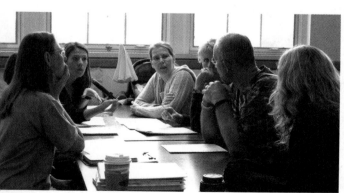

PHOTOS: DANA GOODWIN

local asparagus [roasted in olive oil]." The spears also cropped up on the salad bar and at a field day picnic for parents and children.

Connecting with Cooks and Others

One of the group's first moves was to create a cafeteria "wish list" aimed at minimizing certain items (bacon bits and fake cheese) and incorporating others (whole-wheat bread and more fresh foods). Members sent the list to the school's foodservice director at an opportune time. The council had been approached by Patty Cantrell from the Michigan Land Use Institute (MLUI) about an emerging farm to cafeteria project. Together, they talked with the director — and the spark ignited. "As foodservice staff and cooks began to come to the MLUI-initiated meetings and to what evolved into district-wide farm to cafeteria meetings, it spurred everyone's interest in making change," says Dana. "There was real synergy as we fed off one another." Guests who were invited to meetings also brought more fruitful fodder. For instance, the education and outreach coordinator from the local food coop shared healthy lunch ideas and recipes.

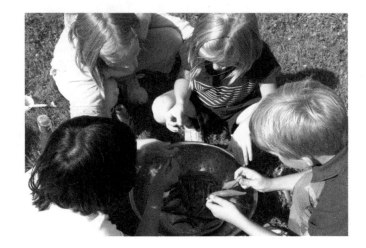

Council members recognized the value of reaching out to parents, too. To that end, they created a list of recommendations for healthy school snack items. These go home via backpack mail to parents before it's their turn to send in a snack for the class. "We now see much more whole grains and good protein, and fewer snacks with trans fats and empty calories," says Dana.

Fresh Farm Harvests Go to School

MLUI's current farm to cafeteria coordinator, Diane Conners, describes the modest beginnings of the pilot program at Central Grade School. Her goal: Find four farmers who could each sell a fresh food item to the school food-service during one week in October. In the end, the growers did more than supply apples, grapes, and potatoes. After all, part of the project's goal — beyond finding new markets for farmers — was to stimulate students' curiosity about fresh foods and the people who grew them. So along with each featured farm item came the grower who produced it. He or she greeted students in the lunch line and spent recess in the courtyard with the garden club, sharing stories, offering wisdom, and answering questions about foods and farms.

As Diane tells it, the day that farmer Jim Bardenhagen bit into one of his raw potatoes in front of a large group, students looked skeptical. But after learning that the humble tubers they'd be served at lunch that day were grown by a neighbor farmer, twice as many as usual opted for the potato bar over pizza. And they weren't disappointed. The young converts thought the local spuds were sweeter than the standard fare. "This showed that kids' palates may be

"The key to successful initiatives is a supportive community in which individuals come together for a common vision in the best interest of children."

— Dana Goodwin, parent and Nutrition Advisory Council cofounder

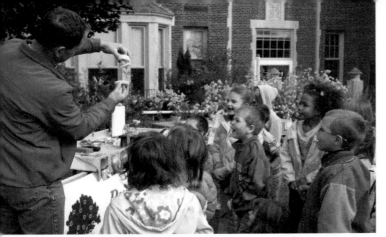

PHOTOS: DANA GOODWIN

more sophisticated than we think," says Diane. "We used baby new potatoes, which are sweeter than the baking versions they're used to eating."

Diane explains that the farmer visits are part of the project's "Three Cs" approach to linking the community, cafeteria, and classroom curricula. Here's how that might work: An apple farmer speaks to a third-grade science class that uses a Michigan Apple Committee curriculum. The grower gears his talk to mesh with the teacher's curriculum goals. Come lunchtime, students find the grower's diced apples in turkey wraps and in a low-sugar dessert. And they get to vote on whether to keep them on the menu.

It's hardly a surprise that students at Central broke records for the volume of apples they ate during the pilot year. And why not? As one student noted, "Baked apples taste like apple pie!" Years later, the alluring aromas wafting down hallways from the lunchroom still reel them in. Says parent and garden volunteer Cori Oakley, "It all smells so delicious — everything from roasted winter squash to cherry crisp — and kids really do recognize the difference."

Each fall, the garden club hosts a festival to celebrate the harvest with the school and local community. The growers whose roots, fruits, stems, and leaves have brought a new punch to lunch are featured guests. The glowing youngsters return the favor by picking their own fresh lettuce, nasturtiums, and other salad fixings, then preparing salad samples for all.

Farm to Cafeteria: Lessons Learned

"It's important to build a program like this slowly," says Diane Conners. "It will take time for schools and farmers to shift their business models." For instance, growers accustomed to large commodity markets may need to rethink delivery systems to sell to a number of small schools.

Cafeteria workers have other hurdles. Preparing fresh foods from scratch requires more time and skill than does heating and serving precut produce from a commercial service. Central Grade School cooks got a leg up. They

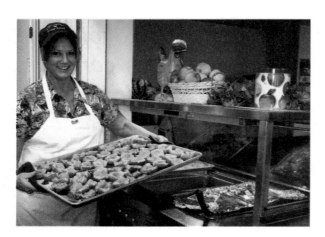

attended a two-day inservice session that featured a local chef. There they acquired knife skills that simplify fresh food preparation, learned how to make healthful soups from scratch, and discovered quick ways to prepare tasty fresh produce, such as roasting pans of vegetables. Leftovers, advised the chef, could be used to top pizza or enhance Mexican dishes.

The Central Grade School pilot project in 2004–2005 proved so successful that the district foodservice expanded sales of local foods to nearly 20 schools. The program continues to grow. Take asparagus. In 2007, the district served it on different days paired with roasted chicken, in stir-fries and wrap sandwiches, roasted, and in salad bars. The 1,200 pounds served more than doubled what the district had bought the previous year. Foodservice dietitian Jodi Jocks credits the repeated exposure to asparagus for boosting students' willingness to try it.

In an effort to inform and inspire similar projects, Diane and the MLUI are creating a regional farm to school Web site. It will feature recipes that have been successful for school cooks; a way for farms and school food buyers to find each other; curriculum and school garden ideas; and a list of local farmers willing to speak in classes, host field trips, and provide local products at wholesale prices for school fundraisers.

Opting for Peas Over Playgrounds

With an eye toward further promoting produce, Dana and volunteer Cori (also a Master Gardener) helped students create an edible section in an existing schoolyard garden. Their goal was fourfold:

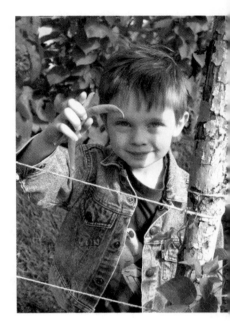

⊛ Entice students to consume fresh snacks in the field and classroom.

⊛ Use the living laboratory as a context for connecting food growing to the science, health, and social studies curriculum.

⊛ Foster an understanding of how the natural world sustains us.

⊛ Promote the environmental and social well-being of the school community.

Impressive vision. But where to fit gardening into a busy school day? The answer was to invite students to dig into the garden during their after-lunch recess. And they did: More than 200 of them coined and joined the Little Green Fingers garden club. Now on any given day, groups of six to 30 come out to plant, prune, or test compost — some of which started as lunchroom leftovers. Together with Cori and other parent volunteers, they explore insects and plant parts, and begin to see relationships between natural processes and their own nutrition. And of course, they nibble, sometimes busting the barriers of long-held beliefs. Refusing a cup of fresh greens with dressing, one boy explained, "I don't eat salad." But tempted to join in when he saw his classmates sampling what they'd grown, he took a cautious taste. "Next thing we knew, he came back for seconds!" says Cori.

The garden laboratory enhances what students are learning in school. The adult volunteers help connect the dots. "We try to extend what teachers are already doing in class and make connections to nutrition benchmarks," says Dana. Beyond that, the team keeps relevant resource books in the libraries — including a farm field trip guide — and sends teachers regular memos about learning opportunities in the garden. Cori and Dana also invite teachers to choose curriculum-related themes and then help them set up plots to bring the ideas to life. Next up: A student-driven edible garden cookbook.

Take Action

FUNDS FROM FARMS

Replace a candy fundraiser with one touting veggies? Central Grade School's Nutrition Advisory Council planted a seed by sending around a list of healthful fundraising options. After all, it's working elsewhere in Michigan! (See Nourishing School Fundraiser, page 52.)

Edible Curriculum

"My fifth-grade social studies program is American history," says teacher Tracy Westerman. "So with help from Cori, we created what we called a New World/Old World garden." The idea was to plant half the garden with foods that were already in America when Christopher Columbus arrived: pumpkins, corn, tomatoes, beans, and sunflowers. The other half would host items that Columbus could have brought here from Europe, such as lettuce and onions. After studying Columbus, fifth graders planted the plot in the spring. The next year's fifth graders harvested the goods and, with help from volunteers, cooked up cultural concoctions. These included Colonial recipes and an Old World/New World pizza, topped with items that originated on each continent.

Finally, students used the food pyramid to analyze the items for nutritional value. "After comparing the diets of Europeans and North Americans before foods went back and forth between the continents, we decided that native people of North America had access to much more healthy diets," says Tracy. "Students wrote about these experiences for our school newspaper and presented their findings to other classes." Another group built on that food and culture theme by raising a circular "three sisters" corn, bean, and squash garden.

"THREE SISTERS" GARDEN

We can't think of a better theme for bringing nutrition, science, and cultural studies to life. This clever planting system, conceived by the Iroquois Indians, features three crops that benefit one another and together nourish the people who plant them. The corn supports bean vines as they grow upward, and the squash covers the soil, helping control weeds and deter animals who might feed on the corn. The beans can convert nitrogen from the air into a form that plants can use. (The nitrogen remaining after the beans are harvested will be available for the corn the following year.) The sisters also complement each other nutritionally. The corn supplies us with carbohydrates, beans contribute protein and vitamins, and squash packs loads of vitamin A.

Advice on Building a Sustainable Program

"The key to successful initiatives is a supportive community in which individuals come together for a common vision in the best interest of children," says Dana. She and Cori advise creating a broad-based Nutrition Advisory Committee that includes representatives from the school community (foodservice, principal, teachers, parents, and custodians) and the broader community (universities, nonprofits, food coops). Identify core volunteers who can help keep it going and help other participants stay engaged. Finally, they say, be sure to pull together materials so you're not reinventing the wheel.

What more? Empower students and families and value their opinions. "If you engage them in the process, you're more likely to see the change come from within," says Dana. "They need to be the ones requesting change." At Central, this includes giving students responsibility for garden decisions, inviting family participation in farm to cafeteria meetings, asking students for input on everything from recipes to raising funds, and publishing the results of students' taste-test votes in the school newspaper.

Involve the custodial staff if you're creating a garden, says Cori. "You need to establish a good relationship before digging beds." Her groups first ran the idea by the district maintenance committee and then by the building staff. Next, they worked together on creating solutions to challenges such as access to water.

Shifting School Food Culture

Middle school teacher Dan Treinis' passion for food education was fueled by garbage. "As a new teacher on lunch duty, I watched in amazement at the sheer amount of trash that was produced," he says. Concerned, he connected with healthful-food-focused parent and artist Bonnie Acker. The pair pondered how to transform school food as it moved both into and out of the cafeteria.

"Separating cafeteria food for compost seemed like a good starting point," says Bonnie. "After all, we figured it could take 25 years to improve school food." But the early compost calculations, it turns out, gave them what they needed to bring edibles to the forefront. The first step was a survey to find out just how much lunch food 700 students in grades K–8 were throwing away. Sure, the total quantity was impressive, but Bonnie was most interested in tracking what students were opting to eat and what they left behind. A group of volunteer parents, teachers, and students kept watch for a week, noting what was left on food trays each day: 54 percent of the mashed potatoes got tossed on Monday, 50 percent of the salad on Tuesday, half the vanilla pudding another day, and so on.

"We told curious students that we cared about their preferences and wanted them to be key players in making decisions about new items," explains Bonnie. She adds that because the ad hoc food group had hard data on consumption, people saw them as more credible. The group also learned that involving parents in the process broadened the base of support for making changes in the school food arena. (Note: Today, the compost program that launched this research diverts up to 80 percent of cafeteria waste from the landfill, and has spread to other schools throughout the district!)

Taste Tests: Thumbs-Up for New Menu Items

Armed with data, an overview of cafeteria consumption, and thoughts on how to slowly integrate some menu changes, the educators began meeting with Doug Davis, the district foodservice

Student Palates Lead the Way

Parents, teachers, foodservice staff, and community partners sit together on a school food council. Students develop and test recipes, survey peers in the cafeteria, and promote "good eats." Project partners help the foodservice staff meet budgets and nutritional needs by using a blend of commodity goods and fresh local products.

Edmunds Middle School Burlington, VT

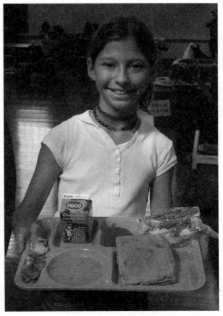

BURLINGTON SCHOOL FOOD PROJECT

director. His bottom line: If you want to change lunchroom food, you've got to ensure that kids will eat the new stuff, and the way to do that is to involve them so they have a stake in the project. And so they do. As often as possible, students' palates are primed for an official cafeteria taste test. Before new items make it to the lunchroom taste-test table, students, chefs, and other community volunteers join foodservice and Vermont FEED (Food Education Every Day) staff to invent recipes using wholesome (and often local) ingredients; classes then test different versions. "When students have a hand in deciding which types and amounts of ingredients should go into something, they have fun and become intellectually and emotionally involved," says Bonnie.

When the school decided to test yogurt fruit parfaits, for example, one class experimented with recipes for the granola topping. Bonnie and the nutrition educator from a local food market gave the group 12 recipe options and

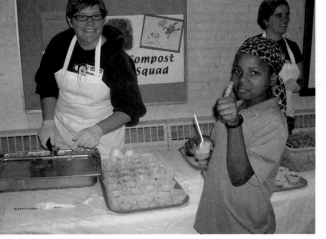

PHOTOS: BURLINGTON SCHOOL
FOOD PROJECT

invited them to experiment with different types of sweeteners (e.g., maple syrup, honey, brown sugar). When a couple of boys asked to strike out on their own, the adults honored their request. Word has it that the extra dose of maple syrup may have gotten their concoction top ranking! The class-endorsed granola now shows up at several schools on the school sandwich/salad bar, in parfaits, and among breakfast choices.

"One of our big recipe successes has been minestrone," says Bonnie. The secret ingredient: pesto, which was initially created by first graders from armloads of basil they'd picked at a community farm. Then there were the 59 trials of whole-grain cookies — many of which were baked or tested by students — that yielded a popular oatmeal/chocolate chip option dubbed "localicious" by one girl. As tasty as they were, they haven't yet passed muster with the foodservice because of the ingredient costs and preparation time. But neither the students nor the foodservice has ruled them out entirely. "If more ingredients were produced in Vermont, we'd love to use them, but we need to stay competitive with the low-cost version of the cookie now being served," says Bonnie.

The Lunchroom Test

Once a healthful kid-friendly recipe bears fruit in one or more classrooms, it is put in front of a larger audience. Each month, a group of students (many of whom build skills through a special "success" class) help prepare taste-test items. Then they serve up the fresh fare at a separate table in the lunchroom. These student researchers go table to table, clipboards in hand, and ask the diners three basic questions: Did you try it? Did you like it? Would you try it again? Finally, they tabulate results. With approval from the diners, foods like the vegetable pizza with partially whole-grain crust, yogurt parfaits with granola, and minestrone have made their way onto the monthly menu.

"The cafeteria is becoming more of a classroom," says Dan. In addition to new student-approved menu items, it sports a sandwich bar with options that include meat, cheese, hummus with pesto, cut vegetables, baby greens, and other products from local sources, and a salad bar offering as many local items as possible. Sometimes farmers participate in a taste test by handing out samples of their fresh vegetables. And the walls are graced with stunning student-painted, larger-than-life panels showing Vermont crops like strawberries and squash. Bonnie contends that any school working on changing food attitudes and behaviors should have artwork in the cafeteria. "I think subliminal advertising does work," she admits.

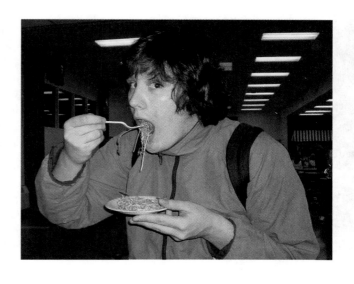

Participating teachers concur that when students are asked for honest feedback and see their preferences incorporated into lunchroom offerings, they become enthusiastic advocates and participants — and cafeteria sales sometimes go up, too. "Kids don't get listened to often enough, or asked for input on solutions to problems," says Bonnie. "But they are excited about being key people in changing a key part of their lives." She adds that they also have a chance to see the relationship between what they do and larger changes in society. "I let them know that their story is being told and is inspiring people nationally."

It Takes a Team

"You don't have to have a degree in anything to begin to build a project like this," says Dan. "There are lots of places to start, and any one will get you moving." In fact, Bonnie suggests that a classroom teacher wanting to explore food education start with just one activity for the year (for example, a parent open house featuring some foods kids have helped prepare). But to launch a comprehensive program, Dan suggests building a team of people who have food in common. "Then appeal to their common sense. After all, kids [perform] better if they eat well. It's a logical link that's hard to argue with."

With that in mind, Dan and other "charter" participants formed a school-wide food committee that includes the foodservice director, foodservice and Vermont FEED staff, teachers, parents, and local chefs and farmers. At lively monthly meetings, the group chooses foods to test in the classrooms and the cafeteria, keeping in mind students' flavor preferences, foodservice staff time, and food costs. The team also invites other people to its meetings, whose input or partnerships can help the taste-test initiative thrive. These include foodservice workers, Americorps volunteers, and university students. Bonnie underscores the importance of engaging volunteers, particularly in the early stages. "You can't just saddle the foodservice by asking them to prepare foods for taste tests," she explains. (Funds raised by the council and community partners go into a "food fund" at a local market, which provides items for the recipe trials.)

Food education leaders across the country echo the same refrain: Involve the foodservice directors and staff, and work toward incremental — not dramatic

> *I'm just an ordinary person who encourages parents and other community people... to work together. By doing this, you can come to wildly successful solutions.*
> — Bonnie Acker, parent volunteer

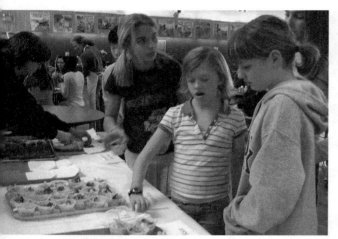

PHOTOS: BURLINGTON SCHOOL
FOOD PROJECT

— changes. "The biggest thing I've learned by working with the people in the foodservice is just how much they are hampered by the government," says Dan. "For instance, they can't just buy or serve whatever they want at any time, and they need to incorporate a lot of government commodity foods." (These are farm surplus foods provided free or at low cost by the government.) What's more, he adds, the foodservice is understaffed, and workers are underpaid.

"The people who make the meals day in and day out are at the heart of school-food change," says Bonnie. From the beginning, the fruitful relationship between foodservice staff and other food advocates has nurtured a wide variety of creative ideas and productive results. "What's kept us working together with open minds is our commitment to the kids," Bonnie reflects. "We respect one another, we groan at the obstacles, we laugh, and we come up with solutions." Groups such as Vermont FEED share resources on topics like sourcing local foods and offer professional development opportunities for school kitchen staff.

> "*After all, kids [perform] better if they eat well. It's a logical link that's hard to argue with.*"
>
> — Dan Treinis,
> Teacher

Menu Tweaks

Changing the menu doesn't mean throwing out old favorites like chicken patties or pizza. Sometimes it means adding new side dishes or shifting ingredients. For instance, students made and sampled whole-grain pizza crusts, which "tested" well. So the foodservice director asked a local owner of a national chain to create a whole-grain crust for the schools. No such luck. But a food company in the Midwest stepped up to deliver crusts made partly with whole-grain flour. The director didn't stop there, and eventually found a local baker to make whole-wheat-crust pies.

When the cafeteria waste study revealed that half the salads prepacked in plastic containers were thrown away, the foodservice challenge was to make healthful greens and vegetables more palatable. A lunchroom salad and sandwich bar now offers students a choice of wholesome local toppings and side dishes. It turns out that because the produce is fresh and flavorful, much less is wasted, so the economics look pretty good, too.

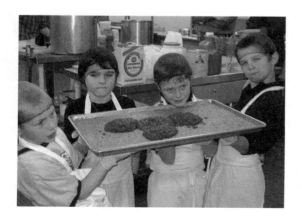

Schools get such a deal on commodity foods that they can hardly meet budgets without them. Unfortunately, say some nutritionists, they're not always the best foods for kids. But Bonnie describes a case in which combining commodities with whole and fresh ingredients makes a big difference. "When Doug asked me and a food coop staffer to experiment with cranberry sauce, I thought, 'It's so high in sugar!'" But combined with apples and topped with oats and sunflower seeds, it makes a flavorful fruit crisp.

The foodservice director and Vermont FEED are also working with state-level commodity program officials to make more local items, such as carrots and winter squash, available to all schools. "After eight years, we managed to get local apples onto the commodity list," exclaims Doug. "There are many other farm products that could be distributed, benefiting both farmers and kids." Through direct farm to school agreements, Burlington schools are receiving more and more in-season crops. For instance, autumn lettuce, baby greens, tomatoes, peppers, and cucumbers make their way into sandwiches and salads. Summer-grown zucchini, basil, and kale are processed and frozen for year-round use.

Reaping Results

"The relationship between our original teacher–parent advocacy group and the foodservice has shifted from one of cautious skepticism to a very good one," says Dan. "I think it's because we all understand where everybody comes from and the limits we all face." Says Family and Consumer Science teacher Ginger Farineau, "Early on, Bonnie and others constantly reinforced what the foodservice director was doing well, and discussed what could be improved. Before long, they were partners. It was the beginning of a real paradigm shift."

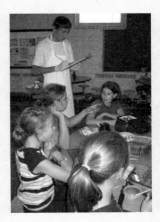

RESOURCES FOR A CITYWIDE EFFORT

According to Doug Davis, the Burlington School District foodservice director, "thousands of pounds of Vermont-grown fruits and vegetables are coming into school cafeterias." Many groups are working to improve city school lunches, boost nutrition education, and build a sustainable local food system. Learn what a coordinated citywide effort looks like:

Burlington Community Food Assessment
www.cedo.ci.burlington.vt.us/legacy/documents_files/
community_food_assessment_2004.pdf

The Burlington School Food Project
www.shelburnefarms.org/PDFs/BSFPNewsletter2005Color.pdf

VT FOOD EDUCATION EVERY DAY (FEED)

Vermont's FEED project is designed to improve food, farm, garden, and nutrition education, and support local growers (and, in turn, the local economy). Rather than simply introduce more healthful foods in the cafeteria, VT FEED's strategy focuses on what it calls the "Three Cs": classroom, cafeteria, and community. School- and community-based leadership teams attend professional development courses and collaborate with project mentors on standards-based curriculum development and assessment.

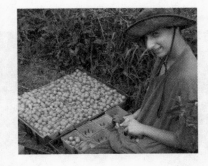

Project staff work with school kitchen managers to integrate fresh foods into lunch programs. Farmers sell food to schools, host student groups, and visit classrooms. Students grow, cook, taste, eat, and explore. And parents and the broader community feast on student fare, concoct new recipes with children at home, and help this ambitious vision bear fruit. For more information and resource links, go to VT FEED's Web site, www.vtfeed.org.

Lunch and Learning from Scratch

Pilot Project Spurs District Change

An intensive pilot project featured a school garden, farm to school education, and a "from scratch" cafeteria kitchen showcasing local foods. Careful evaluation led to replicating core components to the entire district.

Abernethy Elementary School

Portland Public Schools
Portland, OR

When students at Abernethy Elementary School in Portland, Oregon, opt for chard pesto in the lunch line, you have to wonder what change prompted their gusto for green. It started in 1999 at a nearby elementary school. Aiming to connect students to healthful local foods, parent and chef Linda Colwell launched a learning garden and later, a weeklong chefs-in-residence program. (She and the principal found funding through a local community foundation and Slow Food USA.)

When district closures shut that school's doors in 2005, Linda posed the idea of bringing the garden — and an innovative twist on food — to the students' new school (Abernethy). But this time, she thought, why not focus on the whole district rather than on just one school? After all, she reasoned, "to achieve long-term outcomes, change has to come from within the system." She found an ally in Kristy Obbink, the director of the Portland Public Schools (PPS) Nutrition Services.

The women and their nonprofit project collaborators, Portland-based Ecotrust and the Injury Free Coalition for Kids, envisioned an intensive pilot project at Abernethy to integrate the garden, classroom, and lunchroom. The idea was to experiment with new strategies for food procurement, cooking, and education; evaluate the pilot project; and identify elements that could reasonably be rolled out to the entire district. Grant funds enabled Linda and culinary intern James Fowler to set up a "scratch kitchen," replacing packaged reheatable meals with nourishing dishes that had roots closer to home. The pilot project featured a three-pronged approach to wellness: the scratch kitchen, a new school garden (dubbed the Garden of Wonders by a fifth-grade girl), and lessons in a Garden of Wonders classroom.

"I was drawn to this work because I wanted to help students use a culinary lens to view history and to shift their aesthetic perceptions of food,"

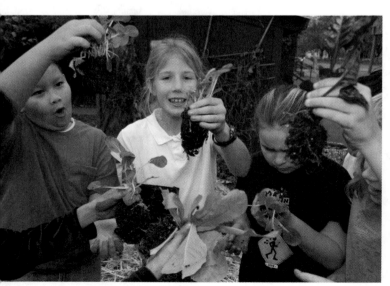

PHOTOS: ALICIA DICKERSON

says James. He now runs Abernethy's scratch kitchen in the fashion laid out during the pilot year. After all, he says, "food is the main way in which family and friends relate to one another." His take is that if students see people in school who really care about food and it's "not simply trucked in and ripped out of plastic," they just might take a second look.

From Garden to Lunchroom

James advocates using a garden as the springboard for a lunchroom program. His reasoning: It's hard to disdain Brussels sprouts that you've raised yourself! Besides, young growers tend to take ownership of the harvest, understand what makes each vegetable special, and carry their new fondness for fresh foods to places beyond the garden.

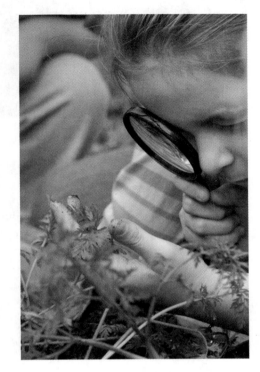

Every day for two weeks, a new group of students come to the Garden of Wonders (GOW) classroom. There, and in the outdoor garden, a full-time Americorps volunteer coordinates hands-on lessons in science, nutrition, and culture. During the pilot year, others helped build the growing/learning link, and now the PTA funds the Americorps worker. A graduate student with expertise in garden-based learning was hired by a project partner to be the school's wellness coordinator. A retired teacher combed through the district's core curriculum and made logical links to the garden. The plot serves as a laboratory for habitat observations, for instance, and a context for probing how explorers survived on the foods they encountered.

But the hottest hook in the GOW classroom just might be the lessons launched through the lens of homegrown edibles. Sure, most kids love carrots, especially ones they've raised themselves. Add to that a glimpse into the vegetable's history (Afghani), past and current cultural connections, agricultural status, and nutritional role. Finally, get kids preparing and snacking on items like carrot halvah — and they're sold. That's the idea behind the "vegetable of the week." When possible, the featured seasonal veggie ends up in the steam table following a clever promotion. Signs like this no longer surprise James' savvy samplers: I'm Louie the Leek and I'll be in your pizza tomorrow!

Other Lunchroom Winners

A growing penchant for produce primes students for other lunchroom makeovers. The trick, says James: Keep and tweak some favorites (e.g., seasonal pizza with low-fat cheese) and showcase new vegetables and fruits that students have come to know, grow, or both. For instance, garden-raised radishes now sit next to other fresh and canned goods on the salad bar. Some new menu items were bound to be crowd pleasers: winter squash, corn, and cheese bake; kale and bacon; and fresh-sliced tomatoes and herbs. But the upbeat buzz about the chard pesto took even the chef by surprise. Principal Tammy Barron credits the students' growing and cooking experiences: "It's not something strange and green. It's something they know about."

> **"I love the food this year... because it is homemade."**
> 2nd grader, Abernethy Elementary School

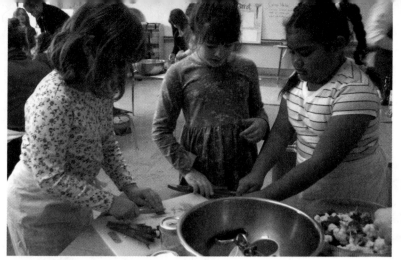

International food themes also spice up trays and pique students' taste buds and cultural curiosity. This year the kids savored flavors of a different continent each month. Once a week, a new country took the spotlight. The Indian tikka masala and the Moroccan chicken with raisins and couscous made the grade with the young food critics — and they were cost-effective, to boot. So now the meals are part of the regular lunch rotation.

Lessons from a Pilot Program

During the pilot year, project partners used surveys and foodservice financials to gather data on the scratch kitchen component. How did students, parents, and the community perceive the changes in the school food environment? Was using local farm produce cost-effective? Would fresh healthful meals prompt students to eat more fruits and vegetables? Here's a glimpse of what they found.

Student acceptance? No question. The lunchroom crowd was enthusiastic about trying and sticking with the homemade, often unfamiliar, lunch items. "I love the food this year ... because it is homemade," said a second grader. A fourth-grade girl enjoyed being given "grown-up" choices. (James concurs that this excitement and openness to new things lasted beyond the pilot year.) Parents noted that kids "got it" about the health value of fresh food and made better food choices at home. The hard numbers reveal that Abernethy students bought school lunch more often than did kids at a control school, and they chose more salad bar fruits and veggies, to boot. Some important role models, their teachers, evidently did the same.

The good financial news was that food costs in the scratch kitchen were somewhat lower than at the control school (94 cents per meal compared to 99 cents). On the downside, labor costs during the startup year were much higher ($2.58 versus 68 cents per meal). Linda points out that this included her consulting time for launching the project. The following year, scratch kitchen labor costs were in a more acceptable range, but still higher than costs in a heat-and-serve operation.

James weighs in on his current efforts to control costs: "I try to save money by being less 'meat-centric' and serving three vegetarian entrées a week." A few parent volunteers help with food preparation, and fourth and fifth graders in a service-learning program serve meals and wash dishes. James also participates in the Harvest of the Month program and gives a healthful facelift to some inexpensive government commodities (e.g., rinsing corn syrup from canned fruit and adding cinnamon for flavor). His homespun dishes also bring in a good return because more teachers opt for them, and they pay higher prices than students.

But, he advises, there may be wisdom in looking beyond the bottom line. "We may not have proved that the model is financially sustainable without

> ***It's hard to disdain Brussels sprouts that you've raised yourself!***
> — James Fowler
> Chef, Abernethy Elementary

outside inputs, but I think we need to study the effects on the kids. Then we can make the case for investing so it can happen on a larger scale."

Small Steps to Institutional Change

The enthusiasm for the Abernethy program was palpable, and the baseline data encouraging. It inspired Kristy, the director of PPS Nutrition Services, to listen carefully to the broader community, which is surrounded by strong farms and a growing number of markets and restaurants that feature local foods. But the conundrum the leaders faced was how to export successful components of an intensive pilot project across a district that serves 23,000 lunches a day. What's more, most schools are equipped only for heat-and-serve meals, and they lack the infusion of funds that helped launch the pilot project. With that backdrop, the project team mused about new ways to define "scratch" cooking. With support from Ecotrust's Food and Farms program, they found an entry point that could nourish both students and the local farm economy.

To boost options for good eats in Portland Public School lunchrooms, cooks began to feature some new kid-tested items (e.g., hummus) and give nutritious tweaks to some old standards. But the centerpiece of change in the PPS school food scene was the Harvest of the Month program. Linda and Ecotrust staff identified area farmers, each of whom could supply a seasonal fruit or vegetable to be served in the 45 elementary schools one day a month.

The debut item — winter squash — raised a dilemma: How to make savory vegetables in kitchens with minimal cooking equipment. The team reasoned that school holding ovens (designed to maintain the temperature of precooked foods) could readily roast items like squash and potatoes. Linda describes another hurdle: "Most kitchen workers probably came to their jobs because food was important to them or they had cooking skills. But in large systems, they're not encouraged to use them." In fact, roasting winter squash was "such a radical idea" that the leaders decided to set up training sessions for kitchen staff. Linda admits that she had some concerns about how some might react to being asked to cook new things. But the idea of working with real food and being gatekeepers of children's health surely had some appeal. In fact, after the first workshop, participants asked, "Could we please take a trip to see the farms?"

Today, PPS students savor side dishes starring apples, peas, asparagus, strawberries, and winter vegetables. As they do so, project collaborators enrich the experience. The Garden of Wonders staff produces farmer profiles, nutrition "bites," and classroom activities that PPS Nutrition Services employees deliver to schools. A nonprofit organization called Growing Gardens starts plots and after-school clubs in buildings that have a high population of students on free or reduced lunch. (Kristy has asked all kitchen managers to incorporate school garden edibles into meals.)

> *"To achieve long-term outcomes, change has to come from within the system."*
> — Linda Colwell, parent and chef

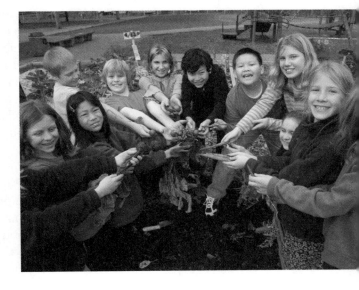

Moving Forward: Tapping Businesses

The cost of the labor and equipment needed to prepare local produce, and the ability to meet demand in large districts, are often-cited challenges of doling out fresh meals in lunchrooms. Some people contend that local food costs are also higher. "I think the underlying issue is that districts must rely on free or low-cost USDA commodity foods or products that are converted into heat-and-serve meals," says Linda. "So a fresh product that is not a commodity is going to cost more."

But the Portland partners are philosophically committed to local products, so they are looking at ways to address these hurdles. One approach is to leverage business connections. For instance, PPS Nutrition Services wants to replace a host of "daily ingredients" with those grown or made closer to home. To that end, they have asked local distribution companies wanting to do business with the district to help identify origins of fresh produce. Ecotrust staff are also talking with other school districts about cooperatively ordering local farm foods.

Thinking beyond single ingredients, Linda hopes to find a source of packaged healthful entrées based on school recipes. Perhaps a local manufacturer would make reasonably priced entrées such as burritos or Japanese bento boxes for the entire district; even better, perhaps PPS Nutrition Services could specify nutritional content and the use of Oregon-grown or Oregon-produced ingredients.

FROM PILOT TO POLICY

What does it take to bring a promising project to an entire district? Strong community support; fiscal soundness; and a deep, sustained commitment from leaders, say community people interviewed for the pilot project. And *that* takes broad-based education about the issues and the promise and potential of shifting the school food environment. But to have teeth over time, policy changes — with funds attached — are critical. At this writing, the Oregon legislature is poised to pass bills to set up a statewide farm to school initiative, give foodservices extra funds for buying state agricultural products, and offer mini grants for school gardens.

See the School Nutrition Association Web site for links to current and pending national legislation related to healthy school meals. Much of it is part of the current Farm Bill: *http://capwiz.com/asfsa/issues/*.

Collaboration Is Key, Change Is Slow

Working with existing systems by building solid relationships, says Linda, is the best way to effect change that will last long after a "champion" has moved on. "No matter how inspired and hardworking one individual is, partnerships are critical." For instance, Ecotrust's commitment to finding farmers for the Harvest of the Month program prompted Kristy to give the project a green light. Just a year later, the leader saw the project as a first step toward a landscape in which school cafeterias are models for health, wellness, and food system sustainability.

Putting a new spin on the popular phrase, Linda adds that it really is a "slow food movement." Making changes in the food system, especially in large districts, is a long process. Projects can surely learn from one another, but in the end, each has unique challenges and must puzzle out locally practical solutions. The good news is that tangible rewards come along the way. Says Linda, "With the right exposure and encouragement, kids will surprise you and eat things you never dreamed they would!"

Food Education Resources

Planning Guides and Toolkits

Changing the Scene: Improving the School Nutrition Environment
www.fns.usda.gov/tn/Resources/changing.html

A guide to local action from USDA's Team Nutrition program. It includes sample materials to help advocates create, promote, and carry out plans.

Rethinking School Lunch
www.ecoliteracy.org/programs/rsl-guide.html

An excellent tool kit for addressing the challenges of improving school lunch, using local food systems as springboards for learning, and linking farms and communities.

School Foods Tool Kit
www.cspinet.org/schoolfoodkit/

This comprehensive planning guide from the Center for Science in the Public Interest is for parents, teachers, and others trying to improve school food and beverages. Includes sample surveys and letters, case studies, advice on influencing decision makers, and more.

School Health Index: A Self-Assessment and Planning Guide
http://apps.nccd.cdc.gov/shi/Static/paper.aspx

A survey-based planning tool and scorecard from the Centers for Disease Control and Prevention. Designed with input from health experts, school staff, parents, and other stakeholders. One module is devoted to nutrition.

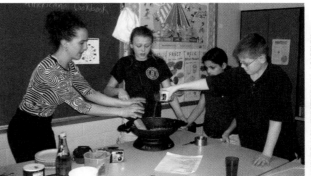

ARIEL DEMAS/HAMPSTEAD HILL ACADEMY/
FOOD STUDIES INSTITUTE

School Nutrition ... by Design
www.cde.ca.gov/re/pn/fd/documents/schnutrtn071206.pdf

From the California Department of Education, a practical tool for creating a healthy school nutrition environment. Features key design principles (e.g., student involvement, teacher professional development) along with related quality indicators and resources.

More Planning Resources and Success Stories

Action for Healthy Kids
www.actionforhealthykids.org/

A wealth of resources on topics ranging from school nutrition education to alternative fundraisers. You can link to initiatives in every state.

A Harvest in Harlem
www.slowfoodusa.org/education/harvest_in_harlem.html

Learn about an inspiring food and nutrition project and download some healthful classroom recipes.

Davis School Program Supports Life-Long Healthy Eating Habits in Children
http://calag.ucop.edu/0404OND/pdfs/healthySchools.pdf

Describes a research study that evaluated the effects of a farm to school initiative, garden, and salad bar program in Davis, California. You can draw from the material to state the case for your own efforts.

Edible Schoolyard
www.edibleschoolyard.org

The much-touted Edible Schoolyard in Berkeley, California, consists of a one-acre organic urban garden, fully equipped kitchen classroom, and related curriculum. The Web site has guidelines, lessons, and other resources for setting up such a project.

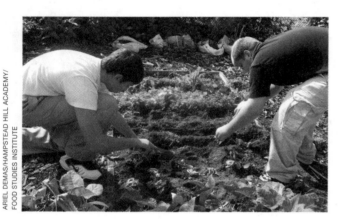

ARIEL DEMAS/HAMPSTEAD HILL ACADEMY/ FOOD STUDIES INSTITUTE

Feeding the Children
www.rethinkingschools.org/archive/20_04/feed204.shtml

This online issue of Rethinking Schools explores the messages students get from the food available in school and from the classroom lessons and barrage of advertisements they consume. It also looks at the politics of the federal school lunch program.

Food Routes
www.foodroutes.org

If you want students to experience foods grown lovingly and locally, or to connect with those who produce them, you can go here for resources and searchable maps of farms, markets, farm stands, and other food sources.

Local Food Dude
http://localfooddude.com/aboutus.aspx

Web site of one-time school chef and current district foodservice director Timothy Cipriano. He is passionate about getting local farm goods into schools and engaging students in creating, sampling, and marketing new dishes to others. Learn more, find recipes, and read his blog.

Lunch Lessons: Changing the Way We Feed Our Children
www.lunchlessons.org/

A respected advocate for changing how and what our kids eat, chef Ann Cooper has transformed school cafeterias into culinary classrooms. In her inspiring and practical book, she dishes up recipes, strategies for parents and school staff, and suggestions for working on local projects and policies.

Making it Happen: School Nutrition Success Stories
http://teamnutrition.usda.gov/Resources/makingithappen.html

Features 32 stories of K–12 schools that improved their school nutrition environments for foods and beverages offered outside federal meal programs.

Slow Food in Schools
http://slowfoodusa.org/education/g2t.html

Describes components of a Slow Food project, including after-school cooking classes and schoolyard gardens. Suggests ways to emphasize the pleasures of taste and create a direct connection between children and their food sources.

SchoolFood Plus
www.foodchange.org/nutrition/schoolfood.html

An impressive collaborative multi-agency effort to improve the eating habits, health, and academics of New York City public school children while getting state agricultural products into cafeterias.

Research and Statistics

Food Is Elementary: Research Summaries
www.foodstudies.org/Results/

Findings from outcomes-based research on schools implementing the Food Studies Institute's curriculum.

Garden-Based Learning: Research That Supports Our Work
www.hort.cornell.edu/gbl/groundwork/researchsupports.html

Links to persuasive arguments and research.

Healthy Youth: Nutrition
www.cdc.gov/healthyyouth/nutrition

This Centers for Disease Control and Prevention (CDC) site has links to data on obesity, young people's eating habits, and related topics that can help you state the case to administrators, partners, and potential funders.

How Farm-to-School Programs Help Kids Eat Healthy
www.kerrcenter.com/farm_to_school/healthy_kids.htm
Research summaries to help you state the case.

Research and Policy Supporting Garden-Based Learning
www.csgn.org/page.php?id=9

The best collection we've found of school-food-related research citations and links.

School Foods Report Card
www.cspinet.org/2007schoolreport.pdf

A 2007 state-by-state evaluation of policies on food and beverage sales in school venues outside the school lunch program.

The Links Between Nutrition and Cognitive Development
www.eecom.net/mfsp/projects_school_links.pdf

Research-based findings excerpted from a document from the Tufts University School of Nutritional Science and Policy.

Farm to School

(also see Foodservice Resources)

Farm-to-Cafeteria Connections
http://agr.wa.gov/Marketing/SmallFarm/102-FarmToCafeteriaConnections-Web.pdf

A planning tool for farmers, foodservices, and nonprofit organizations developing farm to cafe-

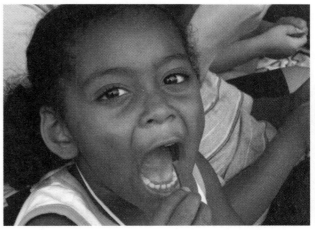

teria programs. Created for Washington State, but useful for many contexts.

Farm to School in the Northeast: Making the Connection for Healthy Kids and Healthy Farms
http://farmtoschool.cce.cornell.edu/content/view/publications.html

A 200-page, user-friendly guide for planning, implementation, and evaluation. Includes tools such as assessment and evaluation forms, sample position announcements, and contracts.

Going Local: Paths to Success for Farm to School Programs
http://departments.oxy.edu/uepi/cfj/publications/goinglocal.pdf

Case studies from several national programs reveal a variety of ways in which such programs can flourish.

National Farm to School Program
www.farmtoschool.org

Features case studies, research results, links to state publications, and policy updates. Learn about the National Farm to School Network, which was launched in 2007, or click on a map to read profiles of programs in your state.

Starting School Gardens and Related Projects

(also see Curricula and Activity Guides)

Health and Nutrition from the Garden
www.kidsgardeningstore.com/21-4042.html

Part of the Junior Master Gardener series, this book is for educators of grades 3–5 who use gardens to teach students about health, nutrition, food safety, and wise decision making.

How to Start a Healthy Food Market
www.thefoodtrust.org/catalog/resource.detail.php?product_id=124

A teacher's guide to setting up a market in which students create, own, and operate fresh fruit and vegetable stands for the school community.

School Garden Materials and Resource Guide
www.csgn.org/pdf/garden_budget.pdf

This planning tool outlines specific building materials, estimated costs, and budgets needed to get a school garden started.

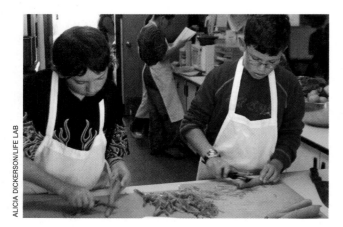

ALICIA DICKERSON/LIFE LAB

Schoolyard Mosaics: Designing Gardens and Habitats
www.kidsgardeningstore.com/11-4508.html

Stories and actual garden plans from the field along with advice on involving students in the planning and design process, building community support, and integrating the project with learning goals.

Steps to a Bountiful Kids' Garden
www.kidsgardeningstore.com/11-4052.html

A how-to guide containing information for launching and sustaining a gardening program for kids: rallying support, recruiting volunteers, developing the garden site, performing maintenance, making curriculum connections, and more.

Foodservice Resources

Alliance for a Healthier Generation
www.healthiergeneration.org/schools.aspx

The American Heart Association and the Clinton Foundation partnered to create a free tool to identify snack and cafeteria foods from companies that meet the alliance's healthy snack guidelines. Click on "Healthy Schools Product Navigator" in the left menu.

Developing School Salad Bars
On the next three Web sites, find facts, figures, and strategies for developing and promoting a school salad bar:

- **How to Develop a Salad Bar for School Lunch Menu Programs**
  http://socialmarketing-nutrition.ucdavis.edu/Downloads/SaladBarDev.PDF

- **The Crunch Lunch Manual (case study and fiscal analysis)**
  www.sarep.ucdavis.edu/cdpp/farmtoschool/crunchlunch32003.pdf

- **A Salad Bar Featuring Organic Choices**
  http://agr.wa.gov/Marketing/SmallFarm/SaladBarOrganicChoices.pdf

Department of Defense Fresh Fruit and Vegetable Program
www.fns.usda.gov/fdd/programs/dod/default.htm

Information on a program designed to increase the amount of fresh U.S.-grown produce in public schools.

Eat Smart — Farm Fresh
www.fns.usda.gov/cnd/Guidance/Farm-to-School-Guidance_12-19-2005.pdf

This guide to buying and selling locally grown produce for school meals tackles subjects such as food procurement and distribution, finding farmers and locally grown food, and planning menus.

Food Is Elementary
www.healthylunches.org/foodre.htm

Features field-tested, healthy, low-cost, multicultural recipes that use commodity ingredients. Includes nutrient contents and cost per serving.

Fruits & Vegetables Galore
www.fns.usda.gov/tn/Resources/fv_galore.html

A tool for school foodservice professionals published by the USDA's Food and Nutrition Service. Has tips on planning, purchasing, preparing, presenting, and promoting fruits and vegetables — and on getting students and teachers on board.

Fruits and Veggies — More Matters
www.fruitsandveggiesmatter.gov/index.html

Learn why they matter, search the recipe database, find snack tips, get the scoop on a new fruit and vegetable each month.

Harvest of the Month
www.harvestofthemonth.com/program-overview.asp

A California-based guide to get students exploring, tasting, and learning about the importance of eating fruits and vegetables. Use it as a model for creating a program in your district or state.

Curricula and Activity Guides
(print and online)

Ag in the Classroom's Teacher Resources
www.agclassroom.org/teacher/lesson.htm

Links to a host of national and state lesson plans related to food, agriculture, health, and geography.

Cooking with Kids (program and curricula)
www.cookingwithkids.net/

Features video clips and sample lessons from an intriguing tasting and cooking project designed to improve school food in Santa Fe, New Mexico.

Discovering the Food System: An Experiential Learning Program for Young and Inquiring Minds
http://foodsys.cce.cornell.edu/

Students explore how nutrition, diet, and food systems are related, and how our everyday choices influence and are influenced by the food system. Then they investigate their own food systems and share findings with the community. Grades 6–12.

Family Cook Productions
www.familycookproductions.com

This organization offers field-tested curricula teaching culinary skills and basic nutrition in a multicultural context. Community leaders and school teams attend trainings in order to use the program and materials in their communities.

French Fries and the Food System: A Year-Round Curriculum Connecting Youth with Farming and Food
www.kidsgardeningstore.com/21-4041.html

Indoor and outdoor seasonal lessons focus on agriculture, local food production, nutrition, and the environment. Based on the Food Project's successful program with teens from diverse backgrounds. Grades 5–12.

Food Is Elementary
www.foodstudies.org/Curriculum/index.htm

An exciting research-based curriculum, complete with recipes, that uses cooperative cooking sessions to teach about food, nutrition, and cultures.

Food Sense CHANGE
http://king.wsu.edu/nutrition/change.htm

A nutrition curriculum enhanced by gardening, cooking, and other hands-on activities. Grades K–5.

LiFE Curriculum Series
www.kidsgardeningstore.com/11-3300.html

An excellent standards-based curriculum series in modules for upper elementary and middle school students. Explores science concepts by investigating food, food systems, health, and personal choices. Developed by educators at Teachers College, Columbia University.

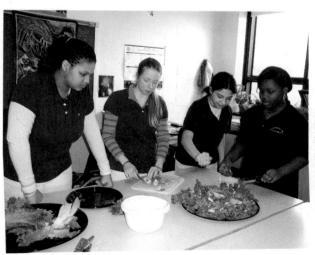

Kids Cook Farm Fresh Foods
www.cde.ca.gov/re/pn/rc/ap/pubcat.aspx

Vegetable by vegetable (and fruit), seasonal recipes and student activities for exploring fresh local produce, nutrition, gardening, and farming. (For California, but recipes and activities are useful elsewhere. Browse under "K to find and order the materials.)

Media-Smart Youth: Eat, Think, and Be Active!
www.nichd.nih.gov/msy/facilitator_toc.htm

An interactive education program in which young people explore the media world and how it can affect their nutrition and health. Ages 11–13.

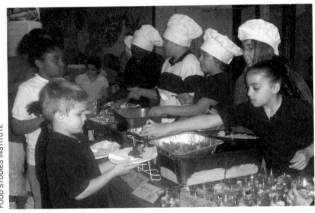

ARIEL DEMAS/HAMPSTEAD HILL ACADEMY/ FOOD STUDIES INSTITUTE

Nutrition to Grow On
www.cde.ca.gov/re/pn/rc/ap/pubcat.aspx

A nine-lesson curriculum that uses multidisciplinary classroom and garden activities to set the stage for students making healthful food choices. (Browse under "N" to find and order the materials.) Grades 4–6.

Nutrition for Kids
http://nutritionforkids.com

A Web site from a dietitian who specializes in children's health. Features news updates, newsletters, and books to help educators use hands-on activities to promote positive ideas about food, fitness, and body image. Grades K–6.

The Growing Classroom
www.kidsgardeningstore.com/11-4017.html

A teacher's manual and curriculum from the award-winning Life Lab program. Features strategies for setting up and promoting hands-on learning in a garden-based science and nutrition program.

Thematic Lessons

Cultivating Taste: Beyond the Food Pyramid
www.kidsgardening.com/Dig/ DigDetail.taf?ID=2090&Type=Art

"Taste education" lessons for the classroom.

Food and Culture: Exploring the Flavors of Your Community
www.kidsgardening.com/growingideas/projects/ oct03/pg1.html

Students explore personal and historical questions about how different groups eat; how they prepare food; and the role of edible fare in celebrations, social lives, and more.

Food Journeys: Discovering That Local Foods Rule
www.kidsregen.org/localfood

Background information and lessons to help students explore their food's journey from farm to table, test fresh fare, and chew on the idea of eating close to home.

Got Nutrition? Rooting Out the Truth in Food Ads
www.kidsgardening.com/themes/food/part3.asp

Lessons challenge students to dig into food ads and packages with a critical eye and then to use persuasive strategies to promote their own nourishing edibles.

Kitchen Science
www.kidsregen.org/kitchenscience

Investigations engage students in uncovering some of the science mysteries behind foods we eat and flavors we experience.